I0569449

Real Food Recovery

If Food Isn't the Answer,
What's the Question?

Jamie Morgan Reno & Paige Alexander

Real Food Recovery:
If Food Isn't the Answer, What's the Question?

Copyright © Jamie Morgan Reno & Paige Alexander (2025)

Paperback ISBN:979-8-89576-084-0
Hardback ISBN: 979-8-89576-085-7

Published by:
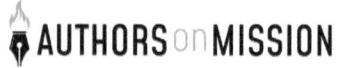

Table of Contents

Foreword to: Real Food Recovery... 5

Introduction 8

    The *Real Food Recovery* Branches of Recovery 13

Chapter 1: Meet The Authors 16

    Jamie's Story 17

    Paige's Story.. 22

    How We Met... 28

    What Is RFR?.. 29

    What About "Addiction"? 30

Chapter 2: The Main Branch: Food.. 32

    Jamie: Confidante, Comforter, Constant Companion 35

    Paige: From the Dessert Diet to Clean in All Circumstances 41

    The RFR Takeaways.. 47

Chapter 3: Sleep: A Successful Day In Recovery Starts The Night Before... 60

    Jamie: Self-Love and The Sleep Crypt 62

    Paige: A Sleepless Night or Two 67

    The RFR Takeaways.. 71

Chapter 4: The Magic Of Movement 77

    Jamie: Movement Is So Much More Than Just Physical 79

    Paige: When Your Body Moves, Your Brain Grooves............................... 85

    The RFR Takeaways.. 90

Chapter 5: Spirituality.. 98

    Jamie: Putting Things In God's Hands 100

    Paige: God On The Inca Trails... 109

    The RFR Takeaways.. 119

Chapter 6: Stress Management in an Emotionally Intelligent Way............. 122

    Jamie: Stress in Mind, Stress in Body 123

    Paige: Power of the Pause 128

    The RFR Takeaways.. 134

Chapter 7: Connection To Self 139

    Jamie: Baggage in the Attic 139

    Paige: Are You Ever Older Than Your First Rejection? 143

    The RFR Takeaways 147

Chapter 8: Connection To Others 150

    Jamie: Boundaries and Detachment 151

    Paige: The Shadow Behind Me 155

    The RFR Takeaways 160

Chapter 9: Mindset 164

    Jamie: What Do You Do With Lemons? 164

    Paige: The Mental Muscle Determines Success 168

    The RFR Takeaways 172

Chapter 10: Bringing It All Together 176

    Jamie: The Power of Community 176

    Paige: Collective Wisdom 180

    Key Takeaways 185

Conclusion 187

Real Food Recovery

Have you ever found yourself trapped in a cycle of overeating, overwhelmed by cravings you can't seem to control? Maybe it started innocently—a second helping here, a quick snack there—but now, the food feels like it's taken charge of your mental landscape, and you just can't get out from under it. If this sounds familiar, you are not alone. Many of us have stumbled onto this path, feeling isolated, ashamed, and powerless against the pull of food.

As an addiction physician specializing in sugar and processed food addiction, I have witnessed firsthand the devastating impact our modern ultra-processed food environment has had on individuals struggling with compulsive eating behaviors. For decades, I've worked tirelessly to help patients break free from the grip of sugar and food addiction, which includes relentless eating and restrictive cycles. I have seen the heartbreaking setbacks: the relapses, the despair, and the maddening yo-yo weight fluctuations. But there is hope. There is a way out. I've also observed incredible transformations—people breaking free from the grip of food obsession and rediscovering their strength, joy, and purpose. I have witnessed recovery from food addiction.

Real Food Recovery is a testament to that journey, that promise of recovery. Jamie Morgan Reno and Paige Alexander have lived through the depths of food addiction and emerged on the other side into recovery. Their stories are raw, honest, and deeply relatable. They've experienced the shame of secret binges, the despair of failed diets, and the physical toll of years spent hating their bodies. But they've also found recovery—real recovery—and this book is their roadmap. This is their story and how they found peace with food.

The stories in Real Food Recovery will likely resonate with many readers who identify as being food addicted. As I read through their manuscript, I found myself nodding in recognition of their stories, so many of which depict familiar patterns of behavior, thought processes, and emotional turmoil, all the hallmarks of food addiction many of us know only too well. Their writing quality is impressive. They capture the essence of each experience, captivating me with their stories. I found their material not only easy to follow but also truly engaging and enjoyable to read.

Their approach aligns perfectly with our current scientific understanding of food addiction. Their emphasis on the "pleasure trap" and the role of processed foods in hijacking our natural reward systems echoes what we see in clinical research. The concept of food as a substance capable of triggering addictive patterns is finally gaining recognition in the medical community. It is articulated well in all the stories they give us.

Throughout these pages, Jamie and Paige explore the roots of food addiction: how our brains are wired to overeat in an environment saturated with hyper-palatable foods; how emotional pain can drive us to seek solace in sugar and fat; and how societal pressures compound our struggles to control our eating behaviors. More importantly, Jamie and Paige provide solutions. They highlight strategies for breaking free from the pleasure trap of processed foods, building a supportive community, and finding peace in your relationship with food.

Jamie and Paige do this by conceptualizing a "Tree of Recovery," a powerful metaphor for growth and healing. Like a sturdy tree spreading its branches to provide shelter and sustenance, they show how each branch can represent a crucial element of healing. For example, their "Sleep" branch explores how poor sleep patterns can exacerbate food cravings and derail recovery efforts. They offer practical strategies for improving sleep hygiene, such as establishing a consistent bedtime routine and creating a sleep-friendly environment.

The "Stress Management" branch takes us into the intricate relationship between stress and food addiction. Jamie and Paige share their personal experiences of using food to cope with stress and provide readers with alternative, more effective stress-reduction techniques like mindfulness meditation and deep breathing exercises.

Their "Movement" branch emphasizes the importance of physical activity in recovery, not just for weight management but for its mood-boosting and craving-reducing effects. They offer accessible exercise options for all fitness levels, from gentle yoga to high-intensity interval training.

The "Spirituality" branch explores how connecting with something greater than oneself can provide strength and purpose in recovery. Whether through traditional religious practices or secular mindfulness, they show how spiritual growth can fill the void that food once occupied.

While there are other books on food addiction recovery, what makes Real Food Recovery particularly valuable is how Jamie and Paige use their shared experience to show step-by-step how recovery can be attained, despite living in a world that seems designed to keep us trapped in destructive eating patterns. As a dedicated addiction professional, I can confidently say this book is a game-changer. It goes beyond food and stopping the food insanity. It's about rediscovering yourself, rebuilding your relationship with food, and finding peace.

Are you ready to begin your journey?

Turn the page. Your transformation starts now.

Vera Tarman, MD
Author of Food Junkies: Recovery from Food Addiction

Introduction

Have you ever found yourself stuck in the cycle where you've just eaten your tenth brownie or third burger, and you're staring at the wrapper, feeling the weight sit like a rock in your stomach while you're drowning in shame, disgust, and powerlessness... knowing that you're going to be doing the same thing again tomorrow, or perhaps next week? Knowing that you don't have control: the food has control, and even though you hate how it makes you feel, you'll give in to it every time the cravings hit. This is the world of food addiction, and you are one among many if this sounds like reality.

Let's be clear here: we are you. What do we mean by that? We mean, simply, that whatever trials you've faced in your difficult journey with food, we've faced them too, perhaps in different shapes and forms, but with just as much hurt and equally raw wounds. We've lived the whole roller-coaster countless times: the torture of the cravings, the guilt of consuming, the horror and sickness afterward. We've listened to the rustle of the wrappers, felt the gut-wrenching hunger even when you're full, that emptiness and need for more, long after satiety has been reached. We've walked in your shoes, felt the tightening waistbands, avoided the scales, and snuck second, third, and fourth helpings. We've been swayed by the siren song of desserts, candies, cakes, burgers, fries, milkshakes, pops, wings...

And we've come out on the other side. If any of that resonated with you, if you feel like you're alone, isolated, and unique—you're not. Hundreds of thousands of people share your story, including us, and there's nothing you could tell us about the path you've walked so far that would shock or horrify us because we've both been at the lowest, darkest points. We don't just know you; we are you.

Many of us who suffer from food addiction feel alone and isolated in our suffering, but almost all of our stories share the same notes, even if played to a different tune. The same feelings have ripped through each of us. We want to help people listen for those chords so that they can start the journey to recovery with a sense of community. We want people out there to recognize that feelings of pain, isolation, grief, guilt, desperation, and self-disgust are shared emotions within this community.

We are Jamie and Paige, two survivors of food addiction. We're now in recovery and have chosen to share our journey with others. You will meet us "fully" in our first chapter, but here we want to give a snapshot of who we were when we were addicted to food, highlighting one very key message for this book: even though our struggles looked completely different from the outside, our symptoms were identical. As an outspoken, tall, dark-haired northeasterner and a petite, blonde midwesterner, one might think we'd never cross paths. One might also assume we'd never have anything in common, never feel the same feelings or endure the same hurts. Different ages, backgrounds, appearances, and paths through life... yet both trapped in the same hell.

Jamie: I always had an obsessive relationship with food and opted for burgers, fries, and other chemical-laden fast food at every opportunity. I could eat enough calories for three people in a single sitting and feel hungry a few hours later. I grew up in an unstable home, a child of divorce and financial strife. I used food for security and comfort whenever I faced stress and grief, which was almost daily. My food patterns were unhealthy from the word "go." In my twenties, after the sudden and tragic loss of my mother, food took over my life. It became everything. It was all that kept me going.

By the time I entered my thirties, I was morbidly obese and facing serious health complications that involved hospitalization. It had a huge impact on my relationships, my jobs, and my life as a woman and would-be mom. I lost my chance at children. I nearly died. I never thought I'd make it to my forties, and, if I did, I was certain it would be a miserable existence. That was the start of my recovery journey... and what a long journey it has been.

Paige: For me, it was sugar that was irresistible, right back to my earliest memories. I couldn't get enough. I used to binge on sugar, eating until everything was gone just to satisfy the cravings. I grew up in a traditional family unit: mother, father, and two sisters. Initially, I modeled the food relationships I saw around me: at dinner, everyone ate a plateful and moved on with the evening; the kitchen closed. In middle school, though, unhealthy habits crept in: bags of Doritos or sleeves of Oreos sneaked upstairs to be devoured in purposeful hushed chews under the covers. I didn't understand why I felt compelled to hide, but somehow, I knew others shouldn't see what I was doing.

It felt dangerous to display this secret, even though I had no language for what was happening. The addiction was rearing its ugly head, and it was going to have me in its claws for a long time. My childlike stick figure started to develop curves, and for the first time, calories were betraying me in an obnoxious way I'd never had to consider before. Even so, the real outer effects didn't become apparent until I hit menopause in my forties. No longer able to out-exercise my calories, I started putting on weight fast, and although I never faced serious health complaints, I was just as out of control. Every thought was obsessed with sugar. It was a drug I'd been hooked on for life.

So, that's us. We are completely different... but exactly the same. We were imprisoned by our food addiction, caught in the pleasure trap. We had no idea our paths would cross and we would one day end up helping others, but here we are and we want you to hear this message: it doesn't matter who you are, where you come from, what food means to you, what traumas you've suffered, what you look like, or what roles you play in life. It doesn't matter if you're a big executive or a stay-at-home mom; it doesn't matter if you're in the US, across the pond, way over in Australia, or elsewhere. It doesn't matter if you're single, married, divorced, black, white, etc. If you have food issues, we see you, we feel you, we know you, we *are* you - just as we saw, felt, knew, and were each other as soon as we met. We all have different stories, and yet they are exactly the same.

This is one of the most remarkable things about food addiction; it is both isolating and inclusive. Neither of us has ever felt so alone as we did in our lowest moments, nor have we felt such understanding and acceptance upon entering a community of those who have been through the same trials. We loved each other before we knew each other because we knew each other's pain. There is such a sense of familiarity, comprehension, and compassion when you meet another person who has suffered the same brutal trauma as you have, and we can assure you that we see you, we understand you, and we love you.

When we met each other via our support group, we both had a sense of immediate knowing. A sense of: I have slept in your bed, I have walked in your shoes, I have been in your head, I have lived your life. That feeling is like a breath of air as you rise out of the isolating prison of food addiction, and it's one that we have experienced again and again through our program; we know and understand every person who joins. We want to share a simple message: we love you because you are us. That love runs deep; we feel it for every individual we work with. It's like hearing a chord struck in the other person when the same chord exists in you. We easily get our 10,000 steps in per day by simply nodding our heads as we listen to others because that understanding is so powerful.

We want to talk to you about our experiences, the losses we suffered, the pain we endured, and ultimately, the solutions we found to free ourselves from the obsession with food, so we could begin our lives anew and end the cycle of suffering. Between us, we have more than 100 years of experience of addiction, and we don't want anybody else to endure the things we endured - isolated, in acute pain, and struggling to break free because we didn't have the tools we needed.

Both of us have felt shame, guilt, anger, loneliness, doubt, and intense grief. If any of that resonates with you, we want to reach out and help you, giving you the information and assistance you need to break the cycle and step out of the pain of food obsession. As you read this book, we hope you feel us reaching out to you the way we both needed someone to reach out to us. We are here for you on a journey that will be hard but renewing. We want to give you back your confidence, your health, your control, and your peace of mind, so that you can live a fulfilling, enjoyable life.

In much of the world today, society has developed an unhealthy narrative around the subject of food, partly resulting from advertising campaigns. Take a moment to imagine walking through downtown or driving along a highway. How many ads do you think you'd see for fast food restaurants, drink deals, and the hottest candy bar or best sharing bag of chips? How many would depict a skinny, healthy individual chowing down on a burger or tossing back milkshakes? No wonder we feel something is wrong with us when this contradictory message is emblazoned across our world.

We are constantly being bombarded with food advertisements and the relentless dialogue that we need to eat more, spoil ourselves, have a treat. At the same time, society has adopted a damaging rhetoric of assigning moral value to food, and by extension, to the person eating it; some foods are "good" and some are "bad," and we should feel guilty for indulging in them. While there certainly are foods that are better for us, and we want to encourage healthy eating, making food about morality can be enormously damaging in a multitude of ways. This confusing, conflicting narrative of "treat yourself but feel guilty about it" has only fueled food issues and introduced more pain into an already difficult situation. It's hypocritical, and it makes life even harder for people who are struggling.

There's no doubt that having a complex relationship with food is common today. Although we've approached this from completely different angles, we've struggled with and intimately understand the problems surrounding food obsession. We think we are uniquely placed to help readers who are dealing with the pain of overeating. We have the first-hand experience, empathy, and understanding to reach out, and we've got the toolkit needed to start the journey of recovery.

We feel that we were brought together by God to build something that could help others. We have both been given a second chance, an opportunity to help others. As a result, we created the Real Food Recovery program and a whole community based around recovery; that's what we want to put you in touch with today.

We based our logo and recovery approach on the age-old "Tree of Life," which is symbolic in several ways. For us, every part of it represents recovery, regrowth, and regeneration. Trees symbolize strength, individuality, calmness, and interconnectivity. Trees are grounded, unswayed by the storms around them, and they represent balance and harmony with nature. For many, trees can also represent rebirth. Each of our tree's branches represents an element of recovery that is key to the journey we're all on.

The *Real Food Recovery* Branches of Recovery

In this book, we're going to explore our "Recovery Tree of Life", boasting 16 branches of recovery that we feel are key to developing a healthy relationship with food. We chose the Tree of Life to represent RFR because we were inspired by its symbolism. In recovery, we plant ourselves in fertile soil. The habits and behaviors we practice each day allow the branches of the recovery tree to grow and flourish. Our sixteen branches are:

- Food Prep
- Daily Movement
- Sleep
- Spirituality
- Stress Management
- Community Connection
- Service to Others
- Self-Talk and Thought Life
- Emotional Awareness
- Integration with My Inner Family
- Personal Values
- Writing Practice
- Education
- Addictive Substances and Processes
- Purpose
- Creativity

These branches are not ordered from most to least important. The order of importance of the branches will be specific to each individual. The first four in the list above are the foundational branches and the most critical to have in place on the recovery journey: Food Prep, Daily Movement, Sleep, and Spirituality. They are the cornerstones of recovery on which the remaining 12 branches are built. For that reason, each of those four branches has its own chapter in the book.

In Chapter 1, we'll discuss our own stories and how we met, examining the differences and similarities that we experienced, and how we were thrown together by chance, or perhaps by something else so that we could begin this journey.

In Chapter 2, we'll take an in-depth look at food issues, why this is our first branch, and our personal experiences. We will explore the problems and then, most importantly, take a solution-based approach to addressing these. You'll get insights from both of us on what food obsession can look like, how it can be overcome, and how you can make a start.

Chapter 3 represents our second branch, sleep. We'll explore how sleep relates to food and why it's so important to the concept of food obsession. We'll also provide practical tips and advice for improving your sleep.

In Chapter 4, we will look at the third branch, which is movement. The connections between exercise and weight are well-recognized, but we'll be taking a science-based approach to understanding how exercise can directly improve your diet, as well as providing guidance on how you can start moving in ways that are safe and conducive to your well-being.

In Chapter 5, we'll be looking at our fourth branch, spirituality. In this chapter, we'll explore how presence of mind and inner peace are fundamental aspects of your journey to recovery. We will provide an inclusive look at how beliefs and spiritualism can equip you with resilience and give you the strength you need. We'll also look at our own experiences with the concept of spiritualism, and invite you to share our journeys.

The remaining chapters will explore the rest of our 16 branches, each one offering insights into our personal trials and developments, and unlocking the tools needed for recovery. With our help, you can reclaim your life, and we'll be with you every step of the way. Struggling with food obsession and food addiction is often a lonely, exhausting journey that feels like it will never end, making you think you will be trapped in this cycle forever - but we're here to tell you that it doesn't have to be that way. We're going to help you make the changes you need to reclaim your life and stop you from feeling alone as you do so.

The fundamental fact is we've both been where you are now. We have our own stories, our battle scars, our victories, and we understand deeply and keenly what you are going through. We'll share important anecdotes, our lowest moments, our greatest triumphs, and the challenges we have taken on - separately and together - to get to the place we are today. We back up our lived experiences with a strong understanding of nutritional science, personal development, and psychology, combining them with our hands-on practice of helping others.

This book is not a long, drawn-out exploration of the things we have been through and the pain we've suffered. It's a survival story and guidebook designed to empower you and give you the skills to begin making changes. We are proud of all we have achieved and now, our mission in life is to help others achieve it, too. Let's make a start!

CHAPTER 1

Meet The Authors

So, who are we? How did we end up here, writing this book? The short version is that we have both battled with food issues from our earliest memories and all the associated baggage and mental health issues. We've struggled, succumbed, and risen up again, and now we are sharing our journeys to help others win this fight.

Suffering from food obsession can feel like drowning. Our world is saturated with food. Our holidays and celebrations revolve around it, our streets are flooded with it, and our psyches are perpetually bombarded with temptations—the sights, sounds, and smells of food. The sizzling of burgers, the aroma of doughnuts and fries, the enticement of "double-stuffed" and "extra cheese," not to mention "whoppers." We are being mentally assaulted by ads begging us to buy more, eat more, and ratchet up the decadence.

Living in this world when food is an obsession for you is like a nightmare, where everywhere you look, you're locked into new struggles as you try to resist, and the food tries to suck you in. Your head is underwater, you're not wearing a life vest, you feel like you're on your own, and no one is coming to save you.

We have reached the point where we've managed to get out of the water and onto a lifeboat. It's been a long, hard journey of many years for both of us, and we don't consider it "over" by any means. We're still in the sea, surrounded by ever-available, constantly advertised food, but we're no longer submerged. We've got ourselves out of the water and we're floating, not having to constantly fight to stay on the surface, not being pushed back under by the next big wave. We've reached the pivot, the moment where we have enough space and presence of mind to look around and ask what we can do for others. How can we get them out of the water and into the lifeboat with us?

In writing this book, we're offering you survival skills and an opportunity to climb onboard the lifeboat of recovery. We want to pull others out of the sucking blackness of the food environment that surrounds us, to rescue them from the bondage that held both of us enslaved for so long, to free them from what we view as psychological torture and seemingly endless suffering. If we can get you out of the water and onto the boat, we'll have succeeded in our goal, and we won't give up until you're there.

As we expressed in the introduction, our own journeys look very different from each other, but both center upon the same linchpin, represent the same dances of fear and obsession, and echo elements of the same struggles in different contexts. With that in mind, we'd now like to share more about our journeys, with the awareness that while they look very different on the surface, there are an awful lot of similarities within. We know that every story of food obsession is different, but in those differences, we believe we can find synergies that will help us all to heal.

Jamie's Story

Throughout a lot of my life, food was my constant companion and often my best and only friend. Through my eyes, food never let me down like people did. I lost many people through death, divorce, fallouts, and moves, so whenever a hole opened up in the fabric of my world, I tried to fill it with food - as did others in my family. I modeled what I saw, and when I grieved, I ate. The punctuation marks of life, both happy and sad, were all adorned with food, and I had a deeply held, false belief that eating helped ease the pain. It often just caused me more pain; I got the cruel comments, the, "Should you really be eating that?" I got the looks and the lectures. Some early hurts set in, like little splinters under my skin.

And then, when I was in my 20s, my mom died. My mother was a champion in my life. She fought for me, gave me a voice when I felt voiceless, looked after me, protected me, and made me feel safe. She was my home, and when I lost her, it was like losing the protector of my world. Back then, I didn't understand that I was my own home. No longer anchored, I found myself out of control, and it wasn't so much a hole I was trying to fill as a gaping void that hurt too much to look at. I sought out anything that could give me a sense of security, and food was the most easily available substance to numb my pain.

I was so depressed, family members were holding interventions, afraid I was suicidal. Perhaps I was, in a way, because I was killing myself with food, even if I didn't realize it at the time. Emotionally immature, longing to feel comfortable and safe in the world again, I ate and ate, and in the next four years, I gained 200 lbs. I tipped from curvy and passable in the eyes of society to morbidly obese.

I want to unfold a picture that I saw almost every day during this time: a drive-thru, with me in my car, feeling totally alone, totally overwhelmed, totally sad, and totally disgusted as I put in an order that was enough to feed three people. I used to spend time endlessly planning, working out how many "forbidden foods" I could get from a single place, like a bakery or a drive-thru, and figuring out how I could hide what I was doing from the server, from my family, from myself.

My strategy was simple: I'd behave as though I was ordering for lots of people. "My husband wants," I'd say, or "She'd like." When I'd collected my haul of sizzling, greasy, chemical-packed food, I'd drive into the parking lot or the nearest neighborhood and eat everything. I thought I was fooling people. I'd dispose of the bags in public garbage cans and move on with a deep sense of shame and sadness gnawing away at me. My depression exponentially grew, and it felt as though food was the only thing I was living for.

I'd go home, and the withdrawal symptoms from all the processed food would kick in just a few hours later, with headaches, irritability, agitation—everything telling me "you need to eat, you need to eat." I thought I was just hungry again, that I somehow needed more food after consuming a whole day's worth of calories in one meal. After all, I could get through an entire box of doughnuts in one sitting! I'd eat while I was driving sometimes, driving with one knee. I was intensely aware of the danger, but I did it anyway. Anything to get my fix.

After eating, I'd be high on adrenaline as the sugar, fat, chemicals and caffeine coursed through my system, leaving me anxious, fidgety, and unable to sit still. It was a horrible state to be in, but what came next was so much worse... the crash. As the junk left my system, I'd find myself exhausted and drained, as though I'd run a marathon or fought in a battle. I'd want to do nothing but shut my eyes and rest. I ached with tiredness.

I never ate like that around others; I was far too self-conscious. When I was with family or friends, I'd carefully watch to see what they ate, gauging what was "acceptable," and I'd mirror it precisely. I put on a good front, encouraging myself to think I was fooling the whole world, when really, I was only fooling myself. I even completed many of life's major milestones during those years; I bought my first home, I got married, I worked out regularly, and I mired all of these happy experiences in thick depression and food.

That's how I spent years, batted between the two extremes of highs and crashes, in a state of constant flux, charging myself up on processed food and hitting the ground full-force when it left my system, only to plunge straight back into that cycle when the cravings hit. Around and around, unable to get off the ride, out of control, and hating myself. I was exhausted and agitated, constantly fluctuating, barely functioning, and it affected every part of my life. I lost jobs, I lost a marriage, and I lost my chance to have children. I even felt as though I had lost myself; I had no clue who I was and felt totally disconnected from the person I saw in the mirror, from the person who ate like she'd never eat again.

I lived in an area where obesity was common, and even there, I was such an outlier that I drew looks and comments, often from total strangers. That same phrase, "Do you really need to eat that?" reared its head again. They'd look in my shopping cart, in my hands, staring and pointing. It reignited those painful splinters from childhood; I felt defenseless, trapped in the mindset of a little girl who was hurting and had lost her mother and just wanted to feel better. I was offended, traumatized. Even comments meant in kindness were so painful to me. "You've got such a pretty face," people would say. It was meant to encourage me, to tell me I could be beautiful if only I'd shed the weight, but it alienated me from my body. Though the excessive cruelty didn't occur daily, the constant criticism and comments were like death by a thousand cuts, and the more I grew, the more the comments burned. They lined up with what I felt about myself, and they were like being doused in acid.

Around 2008 or 2009, more interventions came. The people who cared about me tried to step in, to say that they could see I was suffering and they wanted to help. I was also starting to experience some very serious health complications; I had doctors' visits where scary phrases like "fatty liver" and "high triglyceride" levels were mentioned. I was 33 years old, and already, I was pre-diabetic, with blood pressure through the roof. I was having panic attacks, probably as a result of the chemicals. I thought all of it came down to something broken inside me; I never connected it with the food I was eating. The food was destroying me, but it was also keeping me locked in that cycle, where I desperately needed it, and all I could focus on was getting more of those chemicals so that the withdrawal symptoms would stop. I tried drugs for anxiety and every diet plan out there, but I didn't find what I needed to recover.

I ended up in the emergency room with a panic attack, and that's when things changed. They did a stress test, and the next day, a cardiologist came and asked if anybody had ever talked to me about my heart. They thought my heart wasn't pumping correctly because of a damaged ventricle.

By some miracle, it turned out that they were wrong; there was no damage or blockages, but they made it very clear it couldn't possibly stay that way if I didn't make changes. That thought—that my very heart might stop working—was the push I needed. I looked at myself. "You're 33 years old, Jamie. At this rate, you aren't going to make it to 40."

And I started the uphill battle to heal. I still felt desperately alone. I felt like there was just me in this fight, like I couldn't do it, but if I wanted to live, I had to. In many ways, it truly was a life-or-death struggle, and I chose life. I started seeing a counselor so that I could begin healing from the inside out. These wounds were made over the years of losses and pain. They were what was left of the emotional and psychological pain of an abusive father, a man who had been absent from my life again and again, abandoning me repeatedly. The unfairness of my mother's death seemed sharper than ever when he remained in my life.

To an extent, the knowledge that this was really my only chance to survive made it easier. This wasn't voluntary. This wasn't a challenge I could back away from. Failing here wasn't an option. I had to get better if I wanted to live. Suddenly, it was like having a floor under my feet; there was something solid, something certain that I could push off from, letting me fight my way to the surface and keep my head above the waves.

The counselor helped enormously, although it took almost a year before I got to a place where I could love myself a little bit. I rediscovered what it was like to feel warmth toward my own existence, to reconnect with the virtues and values inherent in who I am. That was the tipping point for me; I wanted to learn how to take better care of this person that maybe I didn't hate and maybe even liked a bit. I connected with a dietician, even though I felt it was too indulgent, as though I was unworthy of her. I went with no intention of immediately starting, and she said to me simply that there was no better time.

After that appointment, my husband and I were due to go out for lunch. He struggled with weight issues, too, and the restaurant we'd chosen wasn't exactly geared up for healthy eating, but we decided to try. And suddenly, we had to learn how to read a menu, at a time when menus were a lot less honest about nutrition, and try to choose meals that were actually okay for us. It was so daunting; I remember looking at the words, weighing up the ingredients, and just wanting to throw the paper down and order everything they had in the building.

I felt a deep sense of loss at the idea of giving up my comfort, the one thing that had stood by me through all the changes and all the pain. Food had been my anchor, with me in my lowest and darkest moments, and I had to let go of that. It was like a whole new kind of loss, and I had no choice but to accept it. I won't say that our meals that day were healthy, but we did our best, and it was the start of a new journey for us. This is when the very thing keeping me imprisoned would become the key to my freedom.

I didn't have the skills to do it alone, however, because what I needed was a sense of calmness and a sense of self, and I didn't have those tools in my life. I didn't have stability or certainty, and I didn't have confidence. I had been taught that love was conditional, that I had to earn it, and that was driving my food obsession. It was serving as a deep wound, and I tried to fill it with anything that I could consume, just to stop feeling empty, just to create some sense of connection and control.

It was only in recovery that I gained the tools I needed. I found a community where I was no longer isolated, where people recognized my struggles, saw me and cared about me. I had been given the gift of freedom, and it was time for me to help others climb out of the hell I'd just left. Now, I want to reach into that blackness and pull others out, too.

Paige's Story

From my earliest memories, I always loved sugar. I can't remember a time when it didn't call out to me – the sweetest treats, the most syrupy beverages, the stickiest cakes. I remember at a church picnic when I was about 9 years old, there was a big tub of ice with soda in it, and I locked on to a grape soda as the sweetest drink on offer. I had to stick my arm deep into the ice-filled trough and rummage for it, but I was fully prepared to risk the pain of frozen fingers, even frostbite, if it just meant I could snag that soda. At that moment, it was the only thing that mattered, even if my fingers ached for ages afterward.

I also remember visiting my grandparents back in the 1960s and 1970s. I can still visualize them hand-churning ice cream, at a time when it took three men to crank the handle. My dad, Uncle Jasper, and Grandpa Jeff would take turns, laughing and teasing each other as they ran out of steam. I watched them strain and struggle, and the only thing on my mind was, "Can't they go any faster?"

Me, my girl cousins, and my sisters would cluster around in our matching nightgowns, letting the cool of the cement tickle our bare feet. Even as a child, that basement utility room had a big impact on me; I remember the drain strategically placed into the floor, just waiting for the melted ice or misplaced fluids from the washer or refrigerator. The missing squares on the circular grate were perfectly uniform, allowing any spillage to flow unencumbered into the vast magic of plumbing. It's almost as if the waste automatically knew where to dispose of itself without thought, like a newborn calf standing on its own, void of instructions. It was a utility room I was immensely familiar with; there stood the refrigerator that held the extra pops, quietly humming in the corner, something I'd identified even at a very young age. It beckoned my attention, reminding me what was on the other side of the white door labeled *Frigidaire* - liquid flavors of every kind. I was dying for the sugar.

It was like a drug to me, a drug that I couldn't get quickly enough. It even ruined my enjoyment of it. I found that I scarcely tasted the first dessert, which should have been a delectable few minutes of pleasure, because my mind was already obsessing over how I could get a second piece, how I could obtain just a bit more sugar, without being judged by those around me. I was always desperate for just another mouthful, to the point that the first mouthful tasted of nothing. It wasn't sweet. It wasn't anything. It was just in the way of more. I was in pain before I ever took my first bite because I already knew how it was going to end and feared the impending fallout, which felt utterly inevitable to me. Eating was suffering, but I desperately wanted to eat.

And I lived like that, on what I consider a "dessert diet" until I hit perimenopause. I knew it was a problem, but it didn't directly affect me for many years; I kept eating the sugar and kept snagging the sweets until I found my figure was changing, and I could barely recognize myself anymore. Gone was my svelte appearance. My body could no longer cope with the extra influx I was piling in. I could no longer out-exercise calories - doggone it!

That hurt my vanity, but it wasn't enough to change me. Not immediately. When I came across sugar, it was like a blanket washed over me, and I couldn't do anything but eat, eat, eat, until it was all gone. I felt like it was the only way to quiet the demons; I had to get my fix, or I might die. It wasn't a case of wanting to stop; it was a case of couldn't stop, no matter the consequences or the humiliation.

I remember at a family dinner once, we'd made Dad's favorite lemon apricot cake with a powdered sugar lemon glaze. I decided I'd just have a taste of the glaze from the top. I wasn't eating cake if I just ate the topper, right? Just a sample. And another sample. And another, and another, and I couldn't stop. I rationalized that if I just ate the top half, it would spare me the calories. Food addiction forces you to make whacked-out negotiations with the devil. I'd bargain anything for sugar.

Half the cake topper was soon gone, and I was staring at an exposed, mangled, naked lemon sponge that looked horribly out of place in the pan. Still, I kept going until my middle sister, Gia, physically removed the pan from my hand

and took it out of my reach. The humiliation burned, and I so desperately wanted her to take it, and yet, I did everything I could to stop her.

And with every binge, I reintroduced the trauma, spiraling into a freefall where I felt as though I was literally being tortured. My mind was entirely split between "don't stop" and "please stop," and every part of me was being ripped in two as I fought with myself, hating myself and hating the sugar that I felt I had to eat no matter what. I was so controlled and accomplished in every other area of my life, I couldn't understand this. I lived a life of order until I didn't. What frightened me most was why this was happening to me; I didn't understand the shift when the demons took over, and I didn't understand why I couldn't stop it.

On another occasion, at a family member's house, I came across the candy jar – all those gleaming, bright wrappers designed just to tempt and tantalize, to draw you in and entice you. It worked. They were speaking to me, engaging in conversations with my brain, encouraging me to reach into the jar. I ate candy after candy and then looked at the wrappers with gut-sinking horror. If I put them in the garbage, they'd know. Where could I hide them? What could I do to conceal this shame?

I remember calculating how much I'd need to starve, how much I'd need to exercise, to undo the damage done. I remember putting on a mask as I set dinner on the table for my family and pretended to be hungry, too. I remember the guilt, heavier in my stomach than any amount of food, and the way I felt as though I was suffocating and starving at the same time.

And it made me feel like such a phony, a fraud. I was so successful, so controlled, in all other aspects of my life – but I couldn't control my food cravings. They controlled me. I felt like a victim. I had no idea when the cravings would strike. When their vice-like grip would creep over me and force me to eat, eat, eat until I felt sick. I was white-knuckling it through every day, terrified that it would start, terrified of losing myself to those dark forces once again.

And when it came, it was all-consuming. There was a drowning sense of panic, a sense that if I didn't eat whatever was in front of me, I would die. There was no space for other thoughts, no room for regret or self-restraint. I entered fight-

or-flight mode, and unless I drove the demons back with sugar, they would kill me. I would have done anything for food— taken a doughnut from the trash, even, because to me, that doughnut might save my life.

I knew losing my figure and looks would invite depression, but that wasn't enough to scare me. I knew health issues would soon follow, but that wasn't enough either. Two grandparents dying of diabetes, one blinded from the disease, wasn't enough. The sugar's grip on my psyche was so deep, the neural pathways were so entrenched, I sometimes felt like nothing could shake them, and the trauma got worse with every bite.

And I felt alone in my journey. None of my friends talked about binge eating. None of my family members were swept up in tidal waves of a crushing, all-encompassing need for sugar. I felt like there was something wrong with me. I had no words to describe the effect food had on me and no understanding of why that might be. I felt broken, flawed, and victimized. I was hiding who I really was.

When I was finally given the words to describe my experiences and to understand what was happening to me, it was like somebody had switched on a light in a room that I hadn't even realized was dark. *Food addiction.* That was the phrase I heard, and I felt as if somebody had thrown me a life ring to pull me out of this ocean. Those words finally told me: this is not your fault. This is a sickness. You can get better.

And I took that spark of hope, fanned it, and turned it into a journey of recovery.

As a crucial part of helping you understand who I am and how I've experienced this journey, I want to tell you about my friend Stephanie. We met in nursing college. She was an extraordinary person; she marched to the beat of her own eccentric drum and walked life her way. She had a daughter in my son's class; she'd already been married and divorced. She was highly active, undertaking triathlons regularly. A zany blonde with incredible looks, she was like a magnet to many, but she suffered more than her share of problems. Mental health issues made it hard for her to complete college; she dropped out of second semester, but did eventually go on to finish the course. It seemed to me that her "picker-outer" was broken when it came to choosing men. She would go on to have another 8 children with various partners, but none of her relationships lasted.

Stephanie was unique in every way; her life was filled with colorful adventures that always seemed on the cusp of outrageous and unbelievable. She was forever laughing. I didn't take her seriously a lot of the time; it was impossible to know what was fact and what was fiction, but she clearly lived for the telling. A few years ago, she developed sepsis and an autoimmune disease, and I never knew how much of what she told me was true. Often, I thought she was glamorizing and embellishing just for the sake of telling a great story.

A few months ago, Stephanie called me rather late on a Wednesday, but I didn't pick up; I wasn't feeling well, and I assumed it was a mistake because she rarely called rather than messaging. To my surprise, she called again an hour later, but I was already in bed. I initially decided she could leave a message and I'd deal with it the next day – but even as that rational thought went through my mind, I found myself hitting the "accept" button.

"I'm just calling to let you know I only have 30 days to live."

I paused. I didn't believe her. I thought that 10 years from now, I'd be looking back on this and chuckling over another of her outrageous tales.

Not this time. She was at KU Medical, and the next day, they were releasing her to die at home. She had gone into Hepatic Renal Syndrome. There was nothing they could do. She didn't want me to read about her in the obituaries and not know what had happened.

We only spoke briefly. I didn't feel the need for a long conversation because I knew we could talk when she got home. I had no words for her except that I was sorry and I loved her; she told me she loved me too. I promised I would visit, though I really didn't want to. If it was true, I didn't know if I could cope, but I would have gone anyway.

I knew she would be traveling the next day, Thursday, so I didn't text her until Friday morning. I never heard back. On Saturday, one of her sons announced on Facebook that she had died peacefully surrounded by her family on Friday morning.

A few months later, I'm still processing and asking all the questions we ask when somebody leaves us: What am I supposed to learn? Could I have done more for her? What did she need from me the last time we spoke? How could I have been a better friend?

Yet all of these questions, serious though they are, pale in significance when I think of the very last thing she said to me. I could almost hear the soft smile on her face as she spoke the words: I'm calm.

Calmness has been at the root of my entire recovery journey. It was the missing piece, the thing I was searching for, the key that would give me back control. When your mind is calm, you don't crave. When you are at peace, you don't need. Calm is the ultimate gift that the universe offers us, and we can't realize our potential until we attain it. To further emphasize the significance of calm, I want to make the bold statement that no one has ever had a binge when they are calm.

To make progress, I had to tap into that elusive space in my brain that I needed so desperately. I was a person with ADD wired with an essentially anxious nature, so finding that place of inner peace didn't come naturally to me. I didn't even know what it was supposed to look like. I spent most of my life in a frenetic, chaotic swirl where my addiction held sway and dictated every move, where I could never focus on anything beyond the attainment of sugar as my first priority, where every moment was the pain of eating or the pain of figuring out how to get my drug of choice. I wanted to get high.

Stephanie's last words to me were a gift, a reassurance that she too had found this place where she could accept and let life wash over her, where she felt no anxiety, no torment, no fear or resentment. She was at peace with death, perhaps the only time she ever found peace in her tumultuous life, and though I am still struggling with grief, knowing that she had reached that place is a greater solace than anything else could have been. She understood that nothing is more meaningful than peace of mind, and she reached it before her illness claimed her. I am unendingly grateful to know that.

Calmness is a recovering person's best ally, and it's calmness that Jamie and I wish to gift to those around us as we help them. We have built a community where we promote peace, tranquility, and certainty in your own ability to weather the storms that rage around you. No matter how the wind blows, you are not afraid because you have a strong sense of yourself and exist outside of the gale, unruffled by its strength. We've created a space that is quiet, renewing, and centered, and we want to help welcome you into that space so that you can find calm, and begin to walk the path of recovery.

How We Met

Jamie: It's very obvious that we both had different paths to walk to end up in recovery and that we are very different people. The short version is that we met in a recovery group and worked together formally for a little while. I had started a YouTube channel to share my story with others. I was considering launching a podcast but had no desire to do it alone. I was praying that somebody would come along who I could partner with on this project... and then Paige texted me to ask if I would, by any chance, like to partner in creating a podcast.

Paige: I had already been trying to get a podcast started with two other people, but one had just dropped out. When I mentioned the possibility of bringing Jamie on board to be the remaining partner, the other person expressed doubt about her ability to commit to the whole project and also dropped out, leaving the two of us to take up the gauntlet together. We make incredible partners, and we believe we were set on this path together so we could help others.

From the moment we agreed to join our efforts, the project has moved at warp speed. The podcast had eight episodes recorded in just two weeks, with 57 episodes completed in less than a year. A community was just a few months later; two recovery programs were built, and this book represents the next step in our partnership. We've had a wonderful, humbling experience in the past few months, learning, growing, and figuring out the most effective and powerful methods for helping others. Our goal is to help anybody who struggles with their food identity find hope, gain the skills they need to stabilize themselves and find their way out of the nightmare they are living in. We don't want anybody to experience this pain for a second longer than is necessary.

We have been given another chance, and with that, we believe the onus of responsibility lies with us. We have the understanding, the tools, and the opportunity to help others, curtailing suffering and offering some breathing space where people can start to recover. Our partnership resulted in *Real Food Recovery*, fondly abbreviated to RFR.

What Is RFR?

RFR is the result of our desire to help others and create resources and tools that will give people who are struggling the lifeline that they need. We spent a long time conceptualizing the project, what it would look like, and what it meant – and its name is reflective of the values we want to embody. The word "Real" refers to the fact that we want to help people start eating unprocessed, whole, healthy foods that will nourish their bodies, minds, and souls to bring them to peace.

In our personal lives, we realized we wanted to eat food that was actual food, food our grandparents would recognize. After all, twinkies don't grow on trees, and we haven't seen any burgers, fries, or cakes up there lately, either.

We set about creating a 16-week course that would turn into our branches of recovery. From there, we built up a community. We put together our website in just one month and set to work, giving people the tools they need to start recovering from the damage today's food narrative is doing to our psyches. We don't just look at food at RFR; we view people's whole lives and pay attention to all aspects of the body and mind. Our goal is to educate and encourage so that people can make decisions that will let them enjoy vitality, longevity, physical and emotional health, and perhaps above all, a sense of calm. We are proud of all that we have achieved so far, of the community we have built, of the people we have helped, and of the impact we have had.

As survivors, we know we have the insight and understanding to change this world for others. We combat the negative and unhealthy dialogues that exist around food and create true change for the people who need us. RFR has evolved from a need, with the work of survivors, and it serves anybody and everybody who is suffering from food addiction. We understand, we recognize, and we want to stop you from feeling alone so that you can begin recovering and reach your potential.

Life shouldn't be a constant struggle, a manic journey of highs and lows, where you're just hanging on and surviving as best you can. Life should be a journey where you make choices that elevate you, bring you joy, and give you a sense of self. We know you can reach this if you can find inner peace, and that's what we are here to offer.

What About "Addiction"?

You may have noticed that both of us used the term "food addiction" in our stories, but we have quite different feelings and perspectives about that phrase. We want to take a moment to share that with you, in part because we want to acknowledge that we don't always agree and that readers are going to feel differently at times, too. We're still sharing the same experiences, even if they take on different hues.

Jamie: The term "addiction" made me angry when I heard it. I was offended by the idea that I could be addicted; I wasn't on drugs, and I wanted to believe I had more control than that word suggested. It distanced me from the idea of getting better, and it alienated me from the community. It made me feel vulnerable and victimized, and I hated and rejected the idea vehemently.

Paige: I was relieved when the words "food addiction" came into my world. Suddenly, I had new language, a way to describe what I was experiencing, and this was a recognized condition. I wasn't alone; other people suffered from this, and it wasn't my fault. It wasn't because I was flawed in some fundamental way. Most importantly, it meant there was a way out, a way to get better. This was a disease that could be cured. I don't think we should fear the word "addiction," even if it's not one that resonates with everybody on this journey. I knew in my chest when I first heard it that it was right cause if that ain't it, then what else could it be?

So, what do we do with those two very different responses, apart from having a fascinating but lengthy discussion about our perspectives? We talked about this for a while and then realized it really doesn't matter. While we need to recognize and respect that the words don't resonate with everyone, ultimately, what's important is how we treat the problem, not what we call it. Whatever its name is, the solution is the same, and we are solution-oriented.

We also want to raise the point that if you are struggling with food addiction, it has one element that is uniquely painful, which few other forms of addiction are likely to encompass: food and food advertisements are everywhere. You can't escape from them, so you're constantly confronted with the source of your pain and always on edge as you try to negotiate around it. Whether it's billboards, work lunches, birthday dinners, or just the food in your refrigerator, the constant presence of food in everyday life makes this fraught with difficulty, whether you see it as an addiction or not.

If you feel like "food addiction" (or any of the other similar terms) isn't right for you, that's okay; you can use any phrase that helps you feel validated and seen. What we're most interested in, though, is how we solve this problem, and that's what we are going to start on in the next chapter. Grab the life ring and hold on tight; we will extend the Real Food Recovery branches and pull you aboard.

CHAPTER 2

The Main Branch: Food

Unsurprisingly, the first branch of our tree and the most fundamental one for all of us on this journey, is food. Food is the ocean around you, but what you choose to swallow and whether you decide to swim in the water or get out onto the boat is key. For most of us, making the right choices every time is hard. Before we get out of the water, it can feel impossible, and even once you're on the lifeboat, you've got to be careful not to tip back in.

The first thing we should do is ask a simple question: What is the purpose of food? What do you think food's role in life is? What role does food currently play in your life?

Before we answer that, let's look at how food is set up in today's society. Figuring out what to eat and when to eat it is a minefield. Advertising is everywhere, and unlike other addictive substances, it's impossible to get away from food because it's a major part of everyday life. To make matters worse, we're directly confronted with the decision of what to eat at least three times a day, sometimes even more. There's no escape from food, and the sugar, fat, and salt-laden substances and chemicals marketed as "food" today are almost impossible to resist.

Before we start talking about our own experiences with food, we want to dive a little deeper into our current food environment. It's been said that if you could step back in time just a few hundred years, you would see a very different menu from the one we are offered now. Junk and addictive foods like chips, fries, burgers, doughnuts, and chicken nuggets would not be found. These *Frankenfoods* are all creations of our modern, industrial age. A few hundred years ago, any calorie-dense concoctions would have been rare occurrences, an occasional treat.

Now, these Frankenfoods have become part of the everyday, and that's a problem because we have very little ability to resist them. They often interact with our bodies in harmful ways. Sugar, found in limited quantities in the natural world, has addictive tendencies because of its ability to release opioids and other positive neurotransmitters, tripping the reward circuits in our brains.

The same is true of foods like cheese, which contains casomorphins. When we eat cheese, the casein is broken down in the stomach to create something known as a peptide opiate - a substance that will bind to the opioid receptors in your brain, producing an opioid effect and effectively giving you a "hit." No wonder it's so hard to resist foods like cheese, especially when we have become used to eating them and especially when we are stressed and seeking ways to relax.

It has also been shown that we suffer from withdrawal symptoms when we stop eating these foods, just as we do from drugs. We should note that not everybody feels this all the time with dairy, but there's no doubt that it has addictive qualities, as do many other ultra-processed foods.

These types of food are irresistible, especially when life becomes stressful; it's particularly tempting to indulge in them due to the dopamine release. Dopamine is often misunderstood; we want to clarify that it isn't merely a result of eating certain foods; it also drives us to seek them out. There's a whole cascade of neurotransmitters that includes dopamine. It compels us to pursue the food, gradually increasing in our systems during this process and then is released in a wave once we acquire the food. It's also just one of many releases that occur when we acquire these kinds of foods: others include endorphins, adrenaline, norepinephrine, and various other neurotransmitters.

Essentially, we want to feel better, so we reach for the things that make us feel better, even if they're actually dangerous and damaging in the long term. It's really no different from other drug addictions, just more socially acceptable and much, much more readily available.

And that brings us to the answer to our earlier question: What is the purpose of food? Although we know that food's job is to nourish our bodies and keep us healthy, most of us aren't really using food for that purpose; we're putting other pressures on it. We use food to numb ourselves, alleviate loneliness, shake off boredom, celebrate the milestones of life, create structure in a day, provide a distraction... the list is long. We place a lot of pressure on food, pushing it to fulfill roles it was never meant to. In doing so, we create negative emotions around food because it wasn't designed for these expectations, and, as a result, it often fails to deliver.

To be clear, if you do this, it's absolutely not your fault. Almost every person in society has turned to food for comfort at some time or another, and there's no question that eating has an impact on your mood. Evolutionarily speaking, having a full stomach was likely to have created a sense of security, satisfaction, and peace (no need to go and hunt for/gather food right now; we have enough). Societally speaking, this is also a lesson that is taught early to many. Who wasn't occasionally offered food as an infant to provide a distraction from tears? Who wasn't taught that good food is part of celebrating? Who wasn't given candy as a reward for good behavior?

These things are not necessarily inherently wrong. We enjoy good food when we're celebrating; we like to relax with a delicious meal at the end of a long day, but it's a slippery slope, and the emotions we attach to food need to be watched carefully. The more dependent you become on food for emotional regulation, stimulation, or any other source of feeling than nourishment, the less stable your life is likely to be. We want to make sure we are building our lives on solid foundations and using food predominantly as a means to give our bodies all the nutrition they need.

At Real Food Recovery, we have a measuring tool to examine whether or not a certain food should be part of your regime. You simply take note when you swallow: does it travel up, or does it travel down? If the food you are eating defies gravity and travels upward directly to the brain, that means the communication to the gut is shut off. Our health depends on the gut and brain talking to one another. When we eat whole, unprocessed, single-ingredient food, there is a lovely "back and forth" between these two command centers, and this direct communication allows satiation signals to pass through. In other words, when we swallow, it obeys gravity and is experienced appropriately in the gut as nature intended.

By contrast, ultra-processed food screams at the brain with the force of a fire hose, putting you in a constant panic to get more: don't stop til you get it; it's an emergency, and you will die without it. Remember, the brain has not evolved to know how to cope with ultra-processed food and dopamine responses, so for many of us, moderation is essentially impossible. These foods are specifically designed for you to react just as you do; consequences be damned.

The funny thing about ultra-processed foods is not only do they have a distinct smell that creates a decadent visual, but they are also often associated with very specific sounds that conjure up images in the brain. Most of us who have suffered from food addiction can hear the uncoiling of cellophane from a mile away, the untwisting of those fanned ends, picturing that undefined but oh-so-desirable thing in the middle. As Jessica Simpson famously said, "I dunno what it is, but I wannn it."

It's not just people, either. Paige's beloved dog Riley, a mutt in every sense of the word, would jump from a dead sleep into full alert mode and do the 100-yard dash down the stairs, skidding across the kitchen floor in a u-turn when she heard the silverware drawer open. Apparently, not only does man suffer from ultra-processed food addiction (PFA), but man's best friend is not immune either.

But it doesn't have to be this way. We can change the narrative by getting out of the water, and it starts with awareness of how we use food. Through our personal stories, we want to show you what food's job is and how it can fail or succeed in that role, depending on how you manage your relationship with it.

Jamie: Confidante, Comforter, Constant Companion

For much of my life, food was a confidante, comforter, and constant companion. Sometimes, it was even helpful, but more often, we shared a dysfunctional, toxic relationship. Very often, food mirrored my relationship with people, including myself; when I didn't love myself, I destroyed my body with food... and when I gradually came to love myself, I found that I was able to nourish myself with food.

I have been told by many family members that even as an infant, I displayed obsessive food-seeking behavior. I nursed for over three years, and as soon as I was in physical control of my body, I would try to nurse as often as I could, crawling under my mom's shirt whenever I had the opportunity. It was so frequent that the pediatrician told my mom that she needed to wear overalls to prevent me from feeding so regularly.

And that taught me, from a young age, that food and comfort were not always available. I had already begun to identify food with comfort, and I felt that if I could get to the food fast enough, I would be able to eat what I needed for comfort before it was taken away. This setup, while perhaps well-intended, left me with a deeply ingrained instinct to eat as much as I could while the food was on offer because this helped me feel secure.

Perhaps amazingly, it is only in recent weeks that I have come to the realization that I have an intense belief that food will be taken away from me and that I don't deserve or can't have the food and the comfort that it represents. This realization taught me why I sought food so voraciously and why I approached food the way I did for such a long time. Food was synonymous with comfort, connection, and love for me, and yet I knew it was readily withdrawn.

This very much reflects the kind of home I grew up in; I got a lot of love from some family members, but there was a lot of conflict, turmoil, and dysfunction in my home, too. With an absentee father who caused drama whenever he was home, my sense of insecurity was strong; I lacked emotional and psychological safety. The only consistency, really, was lack of certainty. Food allowed me to comfort myself and feel peace: it was about me and the food, and it was a predictable, reassuring relationship that I could depend upon.

I also believe that I used food as a Vagus nerve stimulator. The esophagus runs alongside this nerve, and I think I was massaging the nerve as I was eating rather than doing deep breathing, focusing on my body, or using other calming techniques when the stress was hard to handle.

My parents split up when I was around 6 or 7, and after my father remarried, I was promptly expected to accept a new wife on the scene. My brain couldn't cope and couldn't comprehend everything. I remember that time as deeply traumatic, and the effects it had upon me were long-lasting, possibly even permanent. All of these experiences were a major puzzle piece of my evolving food addiction - although not the only piece, of course.

I think that my setup for the lifetime of struggle with food was a combination of environment, what was going on in the social zeitgeist at the time, constant emotional upheaval and uncertainty, and my genetics. I know that my genetics would be enormously coveted if I were in the Stone Age; I'd have survived every famine with flying colors, been a chieftain, and outlived half the tribe. In short, I've got a slow metabolism, I build muscle fast, and I store fat easily. It might have been great in the past, but in today's world, I have to be enormously careful with the food I eat, and that's an increasing problem as I get older.

That was coupled with the hyper-fast growth of the processed food industry, something I think many readers of a similar age will relate to. We were, as children, suddenly confronted with new advertising strategies and brand new processed food options, and we found ourselves dwarfed by an industry that was just ramping up and getting going. Now, while the impacts of this industry are undoubtedly still immensely powerful, society is generally more aware of the health implications, and we have developed some (limited) defense mechanisms against the adverts; we know they are emotionally manipulative, exaggerated, and often as close to lying as they can be without triggering lawsuits. Back then, we had none of that to protect us: we saw the shiny new foods, and we wanted them.

I was a latchkey kid in the 1970s and '80s; I would get home, grab some snacks, plonk down in front of the TV, and watch the cartoons that were interspersed with those irresistible commercials. I remember feeling very connected to the characters in those commercials; they were as much my friends and companions as the characters on the TV were. That's exactly what the companies wanted us to think. The process ended with me at the grocery store with my mom, begging for whatever product I'd last seen on TV.

My mom, a single mom struggling to manage with two kids, often gave in. She knew I was gaining weight, but she didn't know what to do; in the face of a tantrum, she would cave and buy what I wanted just to keep the peace.

These four things—home environment, the social landscape, the emotional upheaval, and my genetics—came together to produce this child and then young woman who could not get out of the water and into the boat. Given the combination of aspects that I faced, I don't believe there was any way for me to avoid what I went through, And this was the case outside my nuclear family, too. I was part of an Italian family where food was the center of every event. It was the thing that the women in our family were esteemed and praised for; it was something that was constantly talked about, constantly prepared for, and it was all under the idea of "we're doing this for the family." From an early age, I knew that food was love, and love was food; my mom made delicious meals as a sign of her love for others, and those connections ran deep.

Our family events centered almost exclusively around food. We got together to eat together. We would spend multiple hours at the table, and then perhaps a hand or two of cards would follow, but nobody cared about the cards; we cared about the food. Interestingly, years on, I have few memories of growing up and those that I do have are intensely focused on meals and moments in touch with food. Eating made me present, engaged me, and apparently made a lasting mark on my brain. Without food, I was barely there.

I was also an enormously picky eater and hated vegetables, and my mom pandered to this; she would make me almost any meal I wanted. This made it much harder for me to escape when the time came; I saw vegetables as a kind of kryptonite. I was literally given processed food because I wouldn't eat what others were eating. I know many people out there will relate to this and to the sideways looks and snide comments from family members who consider you spoiled.

I recall immense shame in those moments, triggered by the family members who thought I should just eat what they ate. I felt, at times, as though they were literally chewing me up and spitting me out. It hurt and made those events stressful and painful a lot of the time. I was the odd man out in my family at the time, and nobody was shy about pointing out my weight, taking food away from me, and trying to stage interventions. It came from a place of love, but it was ostracizing and damaging. I felt unaccepted, unworthy, and alienated, and as though nobody could love me because of my appearance.

Ironically, I remain an enormously picky eater, but for different reasons. Now, it's about health. I still often organize and create my own meals, even in restaurants, but it's about ensuring that I'm eating well at all times rather than the opposite. What's particularly nice about this is that now, my unique diet is a source of strength, and I feel proud of it. I'm using food to nourish myself, not for comfort and companionship.

Finally, I want to talk about my mother's experience with food, which I know has impacted my relationship enormously. I have already mentioned that my mother died when I was 28. She was a severe food addict, and she didn't do the things she needed to do to take care of her health; she suffered every cough and cold, every virus, every ache and pain. By 60, she was preparing to retire and move, and then she got bronchitis. It was controlled at first with meds, and she went back to work, but she had a secondary infection, and sepsis developed. She waited too long, only went to the ER after several days, and then had to wait over 12 hours to be seen. During that time, her treatment window was missed. She died the next morning.

In some ways, it was a "perfect storm" of factors: her own decision to wait, her ill health, the busyness of the ER that day… and although her death was related to bronchitis, the sepsis was from her pancreas, where the infection had settled. Perhaps she was already suffering from diabetes; I don't know. But if septic shock hadn't taken her, I suspect her lifestyle would have complicated her health further as she aged.

The choices that she made around food certainly affected me, but losing her was more impactful than I can describe. I needed her desperately at that time and immediately turned to food as a substitute because I lacked comfort, family, and love. Food was what I had learned to fill those gaps with. I was a thousand miles away from the rest of my family, and it was the only crutch and substitute I could find.

I was using food for all the wrong roles, expecting it to give me more than physical nourishment, asking it to replace what I had lost and stand in for the missing pieces in my heart. It was a setup destined to fail, and cause great heartache as it did. I was essentially asking all the burgers, fries, cakes, and doughnuts to take the place of living, breathing people who loved and supported me. Of course, that could only end in disaster.

It was only later that I found the source of love I actually needed, and I found it didn't necessarily come from another person, place, or thing; it came from inside me. My recovery journey taught me that I was a person worthy of love, and as that fulfilled me, my need to eat decreased. The ragged hole could be filled when I started to learn to value myself, and instead of turning to food as my confidante, my comfort, and my constant companion... I started to embody those things for myself. I started to trust myself, to love myself, and to fill that emptiness with something far more nourishing and wholesome. When that journey began, food began to fall away as my crutch; I found I no longer needed it to feel secure.

A final thought that I want to share is what I learned about the message I was sending when I ate poorly. I was telling my body and myself that they weren't important enough to bother feeding well. Their nourishment didn't matter to me. That message, subtle though it was, was impactful in many ways. It taught me that I wasn't a priority and that I shouldn't bother looking after myself in other ways. It taught me not to worry about taking the time to decompress or to sleep well or to respect when I needed a break. It reduced my confidence and tore down my self-esteem. It said: you don't matter.

And what did I find when I began prioritizing healthy food instead? That message changed. Suddenly, I was sending a different signal: you do matter. You matter enough for me to make the effort to nourish you with healthy, nutrient-dense, high-fiber foods that will satiate you and fulfill all your physical needs.

That message was an important one, soon joined by many others, which you'll see in the coming chapters. You matter enough to sleep well. You matter enough to move responsibly. You matter enough to take care of.

Self-care habits around food translate into self-care in other aspects of your life, too. When you have the self-respect, empathy, and self-love to feed your body well, you start to extend that care to other areas. Up to the point where I learned to respect myself and love myself, I was treating my body without love and without respect - because why would I do anything else? But now, I know better.

Paige: From the Dessert Diet to Clean in All Circumstances

2020 found me, like many others, sitting in a hospital, watching over my husband as he struggled with COVID-19. We spent seven weeks there as he battled with it, and food wove through those moments like a vein. At points, it seemed to be all that was keeping me going.

We would sit in silence for hours, just listening to the clock chase away the minutes, and then the sense of nothingness would be broken up by the arrival of a tray - a meal punctuating the day, giving us relief. As soon as that tray came into the room, I could feel my eyes zero in on it because anything he didn't finish would become options to satisfy my anxiety.

His appetite was poor, and as I helped him with the meal, I'd find myself assessing the different offerings - rolls with butter, desserts, tempting treats - and mentally calculating what would give my brain the most excitement, the most dopamine, the biggest relief from the tension, stress, and even boredom of being. Those trays were like little rewards for fighting through another day, and even though I was already in recovery, I found myself slipping back into old patterns of using food as comfort in these extreme circumstances. Nothing could have prepared me for my world to be turned upside down.

And it was easy to excuse. I was going through a stressful time. Who wouldn't eat poorly in those moments? Everyone gets tossed back into the waters when a storm begins to blow, don't they? Who wouldn't be struggling the way I was?

And then, in 2022, a couple of years further into my recovery journey, I found out who.

Me.

The me that was now well and truly and firmly on the lifeboat. I got to stand up to the greatest trial of my life and found out how using food for nourishment made the whole experience different.

When I think about how to use or not use food, this moment stands out most clearly to me. It was a time when the only thing keeping me in the boat, off my dessert diet, and out of hell was a blue thermal bag that contained my sustenance for the day. I held onto that bag like an anchor and refused to let it go, even when everything else in my life was crumbling.

I remember it clearly. I was sitting in a hospital room under bright strip lights, feeling utterly lost. I couldn't grasp what the nurse was saying because it seemed so at odds with her appearance. Her mouth was so pretty, her lips professionally lined with a shade that complimented her skin, not overstated in the least, flawlessly accentuated by a thin layer of gloss, highlighting her white teeth perfectly. She seemed bizarrely removed from the news she was delivering. "The doctor stopped by and said they will need to take the other leg on Wednesday."

I could feel my body floating up to the ceiling and watching everyone in the room from afar. Strangely, myself included, like I was a mere spectator, unaffected by the goings on, just curious about the commotion. At the same time, the message landed on me with such force that it felt as if two imaginary hands were violently shoving me backward, my knees buckling under me. My stomach felt like that first big drop on a roller coaster.

I remember stumbling backward into my "member of the family" assigned recliner, which had been my safe place these past two weeks. It seemed terribly unfair. Didn't they know it was his birthday? Didn't they realize our second oldest son would be getting married in Palm Springs in a week? Did no one care that we had scheduled a trip to the Grand Canyon and my friend Jennifer and I were supposed to be hiking there that day?

I had meticulously arranged my bedside table with my computer open and at the ready so I could take copious notes of every detail, fearing that my rattled mind would miss something important. Plus, that position allowed me to watch out the window as I listened, my mind somewhere far past their sinking words, hearing only that things looked grim. In every lab value, I heard "plan your husband's funeral," and in every new development, I told myself to start saying goodbye.

It had only been two weeks since my husband was hit with sepsis of the worst kind. Little had we known that March 2022 would begin a 10-week journey in the hospital. I originally thought he had the flu. The morning it all started, he was dressed in his suit and preparing to head downtown to sit on the bench and officiate in the Protection from Abuse court. Practicing law for almost 50 years and specializing in the domestic arena made him a perfect fit for the job. He was fairly new to this court-appointed position when I asked him if I now needed to start calling him Judge Alexander, and he assured me that Your Honor would suffice. Please pass the salt, Your Honor.

That Thursday morning, March 24, 2022, had started in a typical manner. However, oddly, my husband was throwing up in the morning (and believe me, he could win an Academy Award for his dramatics) and stayed home from work. Our youngest daughter, Chelsea, stopped by that night on her way home from work as a pediatric nurse and checked on him, confirming my suspicions that he just had the flu. Even so, I went to bed uneasy that night and found it hard to doze off, something gnawing at me. Only a few hours later, I found myself sitting up in response to a low moan and asking him, "Do I need to call the ambulance?"

Where did that question come from, and why did I even have that thought?

Even in the drama of having him whisked away (I was 12 hours into a bowel prep for a colonoscopy the next morning, so I couldn't go with him), I thought he just needed some fluids and IV antibiotics, and I'd be picking him up after my own procedure. And then, the next morning, I got the call from Chelsea, who had gone to the hospital early since I couldn't be there. "Mom, they need your permission to intubate Dad if necessary."

Wait, what? He has the flu. Don't they know?

No, it wasn't that. His white cell count was too high for the machines to read. We now knew we were dealing with another animal by the name of septic shock - something that globally claims about 11 million lives per year. After I woke up from my procedure, a friend took me to the hospital, and Chelsea met me at the entrance. I remember literally swaying down the hallway, the anesthesia still racing through my veins. When we got to his room in the ICU,

I started crying, saying it didn't even look like him. He was so shrunken up, and his hair had gone completely white in just a few short hours. My daughter took me by the shoulders and spun me 45 degrees. "Mom, that's a little old lady. You're in the wrong room; he's over here." You can't make this stuff up.

And so our journey began, the worst journey of my life. There were many moments when I thought I would lose him. I remember one particularly critical point where he was bleeding and clotting at the same time: Disseminated Intravascular Coagulation (DIC), they call it. I thought for sure that was it, but he miraculously pulled through. Within the first week, his intestines had stopped working from a combination of sepsis, drugs, and immobility; they had to rush him into surgery, fearing a blockage was about to rupture. They said, "Whoever wants to say goodbye, this is the time to do it; we cannot guarantee he will wake up after this." The next week, he would lose his first leg; one week later, the next.

But what had changed in my approach? This time was so much worse than my COVID-19 experience. Sure, I was further along in my journey, but when a doctor bluntly says to you, "Your husband has a 50/50 chance," let me tell you that it would have been very easy to backslide, to dive face-first into sugar and cake just to have *something else* to think about. When you're hearing whispers that your out-of-town kids need to come home when you're texting and calling and sharing updates that the worst of the worst is here … who wants to eat broccoli and kale in those moments? We want *comfort* of any kind, and sugar has always been my comfort.

And that's where my thermal tote came in. Just a blue thermal bag, suddenly slotted into my new normal. And what a strange normal it was. Up at five, I headed outside to say my prayers as I walked around the golf course, watching the sun rise over the beautifully manicured grounds. I marveled as the water glistened on the pond, the stillness only breaking for a momma duck and her ducklings, falling in line, forming a perfectly angled wave, rippling across the water. I stared at these things while waiting for something to change. And then, I walked home to gather up my food for the day into the blue thermal tote, gripping the handle as my source of strength as I set out for the hospital.

What did I fill the tote with? Not chips, not candy, not chocolate bars or junk food. No; many days, it was a baked potato, or sometimes, my own recipe of eggs, oatmeal, fruit, carrots, and walnuts - incidentally, something many of the staff striving to keep my husband alive requested a recipe for. That tote became my toolkit, my very own doctor's bag, filled with the equipment I needed to keep myself healthy through my own version of his crisis, and I needed it as much as he needed their treatment.

I was now living the advice I had given to so many clients: "If ever there was a time in your life to be clear, it is now. Double down on your habits, especially your clean, non-processed food." The advice kept me in my boat, and being there meant my head stayed above water, even through the hardest moments.

We know in addiction that what we are really seeking is comfort, to free ourselves from pain, regardless of consequences. Addiction is an immediate need at an emergency level. It doesn't have the ability to understand long or even short-term consequences; its only job is to provide pleasure, even if it's in a backwards way. It will make us do things we would not ordinarily do, especially when we're stressed. And I was facing the biggest left hook that life had ever landed on me; I had been kicked in the teeth with a vigor I had never known. Now was the time for me to decide who I really was.

Would I let the addiction take over, head to the nearest hospital vending machines, have people bring me fast food, or troll the hallways for what sounded good in the cafeteria that day? Pick up the tray the moment he had finished eating, as before?

No. I refused. I was fully committed, like no other time in my life, to keep it together, and I was "eyes wide open" to the fact that sugary, fried, ultra-processed food would have been the end of me. This time, I didn't turn to food to take the sting out of the insufferable; I gave it the job of nourishing my body and trusted all the rest to my own resilience and my own strength. I knew that this was a time when I couldn't afford to sink into a sugar stupor. I had to stay clear.

I religiously stuck to my routine day, meticulously planning my food in advance, and was comforted by knowing I had my clean food with me as a way to fight the demons that lay in wait for a slip. There was no room for compromise here. For me, that first bite sends me tumbling into the darkest abyss with no return ticket. The stakes were too high to risk even a sniff off track.

As we preach in Real Food Recovery, food and food prep have to be number one; everything else rolls downhill from there. Once you lose yourself in food, it is difficult to be fully present in any other area of life.

When reading *Dopamine Nation* by Anna Lembke, I learned that when you are in the food, you lose your ability to govern with reason and are only operating off the pleasure-pain balance. We often think in society that drug abusers are just trying to get high, looking down on those with such weak volition, when in fact, the real truth is they are just trying to get out of pain. As we fall deeper and deeper into addiction, our reward pathways are down-regulated, leaving us needing more and more to feel the same effects.

As much as I would have liked to escape this reality, even if only for a brief moment, I knew I would not be physically or mentally capable of dealing with even the slightest distraction. Every day was spent begging God for my husband to live another day, then another, then another. I kept telling myself, *If he can make it another 24 hours, maybe we have a chance.*

Focusing on gratitude helped me stay out of the food, although there were many moments I wasn't grateful for. His hands and nose were beginning to turn purple, and I knew if he lost his hands, he would lose his will.

Every night when I went home, I stayed the course of thanking God for all my many blessings before falling asleep. I stuck to my healthy regime as fiercely as if it were the only refuge I had in the world. Food does not solve problems; when used incorrectly, it invites pain, shame, guilt, loneliness, regret, isolation, and an ever-shrinking world.

So, to wrap up my story, what was I really packing in that soft blue thermal insulated bag I carried with me to the hospital every day for weeks? I was filling it with nourishment, the food I needed to get through the day. In doing so, I was giving myself the gift of safety, comfort, compassion, love, peace, harmony, connection to self, concentration, clarity, complete presence, and rational thought. These didn't stem from the food itself but from the fact that I cared enough about myself and my well-being in these moments to eat well and give my body all the nutrition it needed to stand up to this challenge - the greatest of my life.

That's the power I want to give to you. The power to eat well even when you're in a crisis because that's the only way you're going to get through the crisis. It's your lifeline, and you're going to need it when the storms come.

The RFR Takeaways

The Pleasure Trap

Before we get to answers, let's look at The Pleasure Trap, a concept from *The Pleasure Trap* by Doug Lisle, Ph.D. and Alan Goldhamer, D.C., who explored humans' relationship with diet and how this affects our health. Essentially, they theorized that people have a biological tendency to seek high-calorie foods because this aided our survival way back in our evolutionary past. These foods would have the most value, helping to protect us from starvation in times of food scarcity. The higher in calories the food, the more value it would have held. Bear in mind that the biggest nutritional threat we would have faced in our evolutionary history was starvation - not diabetes, heart disease, etc.

Equally, foods that can be obtained with minimal effort on our part would have been of particular value. If we don't have to expend energy looking for them, they're a preferable source of nutrition because they again increase survival chances and help us survive periods of food scarcity.

This is the world we evolved in—a world where calorie-rich, low-effort foods were far more likely to ensure our survival. It means we have an instinctive preference for foods rich in calories, and also that we don't really enjoy exercising very much – in the past, it wouldn't have had any major advantages. Calorically dense foods tend to be those rich in sugar and fat, and these are the ones that generally trigger pleasure signals, reinforcing our instinct to find and consume them. The higher the calories and the lower the effort, the more enticing the food is... no wonder we turn to processed food and drive-thrus!

Unfortunately, it's not just the writers of *The Pleasure Trap* who have come to this understanding: the food industry knows it too. They design foods to tap into those reward signals, making meals and snacks that are essentially irresistible on a biological level. They have been doing this for many years – how many advertisements can you think of that have something about irresistibleness in them? Take Lay's Potato Chips, for example: "Betcha can't eat just one." We all know that slogan, which has been around since the 1960s, and it's absolutely true!

Food companies are so aware of the power this has that they employ scientists specifically to drive up the irresistible quality of their products. Initially, they just focused on flavors, but these days, they use addictive chemicals that we simply can't get enough of. Take MSG, for example; this has been used to enhance the flavor of our foods since the 1950s, and it causes an increased appetite and reduced satiety signals. Many of the foods we eat are similarly engineered so that we eat more than we need to; they manipulate our predilection for high-fat, high-sugar options and bypass our natural signals. They aren't designed for nourishment; they are designed to be irresistible. They are designed to promote misuse.

Unfortunately, the industry has also focused on constant availability, something that the internet and online ordering have only added to. Whether it's from your nearest grocery store or fast food restaurant, you can generally get almost any kind of high-calorie food without going much out of your way and often without leaving your house. However, our minds haven't had a chance to adapt to this world yet; we are still hardwired to cope with famines and scarcities. We shouldn't be able to obtain high-calorie foods just anywhere, with no physical effort. This is why we now see a plethora of hyper-attractive, artificial foods dominating the market and why we're seeing diabetes, heart disease, and cancer skyrocketing. Sadly, humans simply aren't meant to exist in a world filled with McDonald's and Pizza Huts.

Humans are hard-wired to seek a diet rich in calories, but in today's world, that drive is a major problem. We simply don't have the inbuilt processes to control these urges, which means we have to work a lot harder to stay ahead of them.

This is what Lisle and Goldhamer termed "The Pleasure Trap," a world where we are trapped in the pleasure responses of high-calorie foods.

We want to note that The Pleasure Trap impacts slim individuals, too; we are all geared to respond to food in this way. Many people who manage to maintain a healthy weight aren't doing so because of discipline (though, of course, some are) but because they have faster metabolisms and more sensitive satiety mechanisms, meaning that they eat less overall. However, they are still vulnerable to these high-calorie foods, even if they don't realize it.

Of course, the real question is, how do we get out of this trap? The good news is that identifying The Pleasure Trap is the first key step. Once you know that you're hardwired to seek calories and that the modern world is at odds with this evolutionary trait, you can start making conscious efforts to short-circuit and subvert the process that draws you toward unhealthy foods.

As you start doing this more frequently and thinking about your food in new ways, you will find it easier and easier to resist The Pleasure Trap. You will begin to see food not as a means to keep hunger at bay or make yourself feel good but to nourish your body, making it easier to take your choices seriously.

Furthermore, since many of the foods in question are addictive or have addictive properties, your desire to eat them will gradually decrease. It's like quitting any drug: hard at first (often exceptionally so), but easier with every step in the right direction.

One practical way to approach getting out of The Pleasure Trap is to avoid buying calorically dense foods at all; you can't give in to your cravings if they aren't in your house. Instead, find foods you enjoy that are nutrient-dense and stock up on these. If you've only got healthy foods at your disposal, these are what you will turn to when hunger hits!

We also wouldn't recommend waiting until you're really hungry to eat. While it might seem a good way to reduce your overall food intake, being really hungry often leads people to overcompensate and eat too much. Regular, filling meals can be a more effective way of losing weight, provided you choose healthy options. As your body adapts and the withdrawal symptoms from processed food fade, you'll find that healthier options become more appetizing and enjoyable.

Once your taste buds have "rebooted," your appreciation for single-ingredient, natural, whole foods and their rich flavors and textures will grow. It takes time for this acclimatization to occur, but there are significant benefits in terms of your energy levels, your vitality, and your overall health and well-being, and it can all be achieved without sacrificing your enjoyment of food.

Bear in mind that it's rare for foods to be both calorie-dense and nutrient-dense, so you're generally choosing one or the other. Of course, no foods provide all the nutrients we need, so we depend upon a varied diet with plenty of fresh ingredients and minimally processed foods. Fruits and vegetables are at the top of this list and are low in calories. Fish, lean meats, whole grains, legumes, nuts, seeds, and dairy are also high in nutrients. However, if you find dairy triggers overconsumption and loss of control, it's best to find the nutrition you need from calming sources.

The Ego Trap

To go with The Pleasure Trap, we also need to understand The Ego Trap, a second theory created by Lisle and Goldhamer. Understanding this trap is critical for fixing food issues and dealing with the psychology behind overeating.

To briefly define it, your ego is your conscious self. It can feed into your sense of self-importance, and it reflects the image of your ideal self (often modeled on other people you know), as well as the standards you want to fulfill. However, the ego can also be a negative influence, triggering problems and making your life harder.

Your ego often generates your expectations about how something is going to go and can, therefore, set you up to fail at times. It will frequently self-handicap and self-sabotage because this feeds into a subconscious desire to avoid being judged... and we can't be judged if we aren't doing our best, right? The ego attempts to shift blame to the external world rather than allowing it to fall on us.

We often don't realize that we are self-sabotaging (and indeed, think we are trying our best), but the ego is setting us up to fail because it doesn't want to face the realization that we might try our best and still fail. It's much better to put in minimal effort so that the failure can be excused. We see this in many areas of life. Have you ever found yourself goofing off when you should have been studying? Or staying up late the night before a big work presentation so you have an excuse to do badly? Sadly, this is what The Ego Trap leads to, and it plays a major role in food and dieting.

If you sabotage yourself with valid excuses to fail, you don't have to face the fact you failed because you've got external reasons for it. Your ego is all about defense mechanisms that will protect you and your sense of self, and it will use these shamelessly when it comes to diet. You're extra tired today, or it's been a hard week at work, or you did well at X, so you deserve a treat, or you'll just have a few bites of cake because it's a celebration. The excuses are endless.

Whenever we take up a challenge in life, our egos kick in and start impacting how we view the situation. If, for example, you tell others you are planning to lose weight, you are at risk of stepping into The Ego Trap. You are setting yourself up to fail, but at the same time, everybody else is expecting you to succeed. Remember, many people aren't aware of The Pleasure Trap and believe that they can moderate processed foods to a healthy level. That means they think it will be easy for you to give up unhealthy foods because they think they are able to do so without much difficulty. This puts you in a difficult situation where you are keen to self-sabotage, and the expectations of others are very high.

Humans care immensely about what other people think about them because we are used to being dependent on the approval of the group for our very survival. That means that you feel ashamed when you don't achieve your goals, and others judge you, even if this judgment is only perceived rather than real. Setting a high goal will unfortunately put you in precisely this position, where your ego stops you from trying, and others fail to understand why it is so hard for you. We think that if we can't do it all, we won't do it *at all*. We don't focus on what we've done well and the possibility of doing even better in the future.

So, what's the answer? Well, identifying when your ego is sabotaging you is an excellent start because it will help you mitigate this sabotage. You can also break big goals down into small goals, which are more achievable. If you want to stop eating at drive-thrus, for example, you might decide that you are initially going to cut down to once or twice per week, and then once or twice every two weeks, and so on. Smaller goals can feel more achievable, and means you are more likely to actually undertake them.

Another effective strategy is to increase the cost-benefit assessment and reduce the challenge that you're setting for yourself if you're struggling. Although you might still have a goal of 100% healthy eating, sometimes you may decide to aim for 80% instead. This will allow you to celebrate all your progress rather than feeling like a failure over that last 20%. Remember, 80% is so much better than 0%! Even 20% is better than 0%.

Remember, too, that you're often doing a lot better than you think. Years ago, we worked with a client who had just come back from vacation in Mexico and was devastated that she'd eaten out far more than she intended. "I had great intentions, but when you're looking at salads, and you're looking at hot fries by the ocean... I just failed."

She was devastated. It ruined her vacation and her first days back. She was so upset with herself, so guilt-ridden, so disappointed and discouraged that we were astonished by how hard she was on herself (even though, yes, we have definitely been there). So we asked her, "Well, how many meals did you have, and how many times did you miss your goal?"

She thought about it a bit. "I had ten meals, and three were off-track."

Three meals. That was what she was destroying her happy vacation memories and tearing herself down for. In her misery, she was missing the fact that 70% of her meals had been on track, and that was 70% better than her last vacation! We sat and talked about it together, and it was a lesson for all three of us in progress over perfection. We all need to focus on the improvement and the gains, not the times when we miss. As Paige put it in that conversation, 90% is still an A, and at 70%, you're still passing! A lot of us forget that.

This approach will help your self-esteem and make you feel more positive about dieting, increasing your confidence in yourself and your ability to achieve. It will also make dieting a much more pleasant and less stressful process; if you're constantly berating yourself for failing, you'll give up sooner rather than later – but if you celebrate every pound lost, you'll find you've got much more staying power.

In short, be kind and positive about dieting, and you'll thwart The Ego Trap and give yourself greatly improved chances of success when it comes to weight loss. You will also find that your sense of peace and satisfaction is greatly improved if you don't constantly trip yourself up and then feel guilty about it.

The Goal of Abstinence: Is it Realistic?

Today is not a world that knows abstinence. It's a world that encourages gluttony. It's a world where we feast, glorifying in ever-bigger cakes, more generous layers of frosting, double-cheese and extra-stuffed crusts... until we are extra-stuffed ourselves.

Many of us are positively drowning in food, and it's impossible to escape from it. When was the last time you celebrated a birthday party without cake? We had one of our members tell us that they literally didn't know how to get through their birthday party without a cake, so deeply ingrained and internalized is this need for the reward, the drug, the food. These events are the exclamation marks of life, but without the food, it can feel as though they are nothing but periods. There's no bang, no flash.

This is the world we are being asked to live in and recover in, and it's a painful one. Our lives are geared exclusively around the next bite, and at times, food is positively shoved down our throats until we are choking, from morning to night. It's everywhere, on everything. Check your devices - you'll see news, sports, celebrities, and... recipes.

We know people who have certain restaurants on their bucket lists. When you step back and look at that objectively, it's staggering. On a list of the things you want to do before you die, is eating in one particular restaurant important enough to make the cut? This is the world that advertising and junk food have created, and it's the one we have to get out of, even though that often means getting out of the water entirely.

If you're looking for a halfway house, a midpoint that means you can enjoy your burgers, fries, sodas and milkshakes without impacting your health... we hate to say it, but this doesn't exist for most people. There's no way to stay in the lifeboat and swim in the sea. Abstinence is not the path most people are looking for, but it is the one we know works. If you're on the extreme side of addiction, moderation is often not the answer; abstinence is.

Many of us start this journey in a bargaining position. We look for moderation and compromises. We want our drug of choice, and we also want calmness, a good figure, no cravings, and so on but the more you walk this path, the more you realize that there is no middle option for those of us who suffer from food addiction. You can't just have a bit of that drug. Our world is too heavily saturated in food. You will be constantly under fire, clobbered by society, by the media, by the adverts - everything telling you to make use of that constant availability and eat, eat, eat.

Trying to moderate will put you in a place of constant hell, where you are always bargaining, pleading, calculating, and wanting. It feels as though you're constantly denying yourself, and it's ten times worse than a world in which you *do* constantly deny yourself because if you take these foods off the table, there's no argument and no temptation. It simply isn't an option. All of that pleading with yourself, the guilt, the anguish, the longing... it falls away, and you can live burden-free.

A world where you aren't constantly tempted is a world in which you can breathe more freely, and everything becomes simple. You don't have to wonder whether you've done enough exercise to earn a sliver of cake or been "good enough" to stop by a drive-thru. You cut these experiences out altogether, and you stop longing for them. You'll no longer be playing tug-of-war with your two desires, the desire for food and the desire for health. You'll have chosen health, and you'll fall firmly in this camp, where you can find peace. The fight is over, and health has won.

If you're currently thinking, "I can't. It's not possible. I'm just not strong enough," let us assure you that we've been there, our community has been there, and we get it. We know the panic, fear, and sense of loss that earmarks the start of this journey. We also know how unfair these moments are. The world blames you for struggling with the very situation that it has instigated, and many of us feel like we're at fault for not being strong enough to deal with this.

All of that blame lifts away when you make the choice of abstinence. It might feel at first like you're losing something, but we promise that what you will be gaining is control and a sense of respect for your body that will nourish you even in your darkest, most difficult moments.

When you make healthy choices, you send a simple message to yourself every single time you do it. You are telling your body, "I care about you enough to give you the nourishment you need. I love you enough to feed you well because you are inherently valuable, and you are loved."

That message is empowering, reassuring, and calming. It will get you through the hard moments when you feel like you simply can't do it because it reaffirms your worth and your sense of inner value.

However, remember The Ego Trap. "If I can't do it all, I won't do it *at all*." That's not helpful. That's why we want to build on this idea of abstinence; we don't want to say, "You can never have a bite; you have failed if you slip." None of us wants to think that we can never again have a bite of cake, a sip of soda, a fry or two, and that kind of extremist thinking is likely to send you over the edge and put you back at square one.

That's why here, we're going to voice a somewhat unusual stance: it's okay to make mistakes. Most people slip sometimes, and we want to stress very clearly that the world does not end. We have to be realistic; we can aim for abstinence most of the time and recognize that sometimes, we're going to miss it. Forgive yourself when it happens, and look to the future.

That latter part is critical. What comes next?

It's about those moments after the abstinence has gone wrong, and you're sitting with a sinking feeling of guilt, failure, and judgment. We want you to take those moments and turn them into something else. Not "Why did I do that?" or "How can I ever get past this?" but "What can I learn from this?" and "What's my game plan now?"

We all slip sometimes. Is it realistic to think that we will abstain from these foods for our entire lives? It's a nice thought, and it's what we should aim for, but we also have to realize that if this black-and-white thinking is causing pain, it's not helping. Being set up for shame and guilt because you occasionally slip off the lifeboat and into the water doesn't help. All you need to do is focus on how you will get back on the boat without judgment, without fear, without reproach.

In the bigger picture, a bite of cake, a bag of chips, a burger and fries, none of these things truly matter. They aren't going to kill you. What matters is that you get back out of the water and onto the boat, and you're going to be far more capable of doing that if you don't beat yourself up for falling off in the first place. The waves are rocky, and the pull of the ocean is immensely strong. Focus your energies on getting back aboard, and it will be okay. You can spend energy beating yourself up and feeling guilty, or you can use the same energy to make a plan and move forward. At RFR, we focus on compassion and the message that you never fail as long as you keep trying. We're an action-oriented community and we concentrate on what action we can take, rather than spending energy on perceived losses.

It's also important to be aware that this is different for everybody. We're not advocating people plunge into the ocean again whenever they feel like it, and we recognize that it can be a slippery slope... but we also recognize that all-or-nothing thinking, reproachfulness, and guilt about mistakes is harmful. *We all make mistakes*, and it's a crucial part of recovery to remember this. We've been there in those after-moments, the guilt and misery, the wishing you could undo, and we don't want the rock bottom that comes with these moments to be a place of judgment. We'd rather you had a soft landing so you can pick yourself up and get back on track as soon as possible.

For both of us, we hope very much that we can stay on our paths and uphold our choices, but we also want to recognize that the food environment we live in is constantly trying to pull us back into the water and that the best way to deal with slip-ups when they occur is to practice self-compassion and an understanding of just how difficult this space is. After all, no one has ever hated themselves into recovery.

These moments are learning opportunities, too; you've got a chance to assess the waves and your position on the boat, figure out what caused you to go overboard, and determine what might help you stay on next time. This process lets you turn guilt into something far more useful: learning.

However, we recognize that this is a potentially slippery slope and needs to be treated with care. For that reason, we came up with this measure: calm is a barometer of where you are.

For those who would like to moderate and believe they can walk this line, we'd like to give you a simple question that you can use to determine whether you are capable of this or not.

Are you still at peace?

Can you eat a slice of cake and move on, enjoy the day, and have fun? Or will you spiral into regret or obsession, constantly returning for more, hating yourself for what you did?

Try this question on yourself the next time you consider abstinence versus indulgence. Use your sense of inner peace as a barometer for where you are. If you can occasionally eat something without cravings and without regret, you may be in a position to manage moderation. We don't care if people sometimes eat processed, unhealthy foods as long as it's not creating a cascade and it's not disrupting their equilibrium. If the cake, chips, burger, etc., is going to cause you grief, then you're not in a place where you should give in. Similarly, if you are using these foods and depending on them to fill spaces in your life, you shouldn't give in.

It's totally okay not to be in a place where you can give in; we are both in this place, especially with some foods. There are simply some things that we cannot eat one bite of and walk away, so we choose abstinence, and we stay in the boat most of the time. We also give in and indulge in other foods occasionally when we know that we're using them in healthy and controllable ways.

Essentially, it's okay to say "Yes, I can" sometimes and "No, I can't" other times. You just have to recognize what feels right to you, how much pain food is causing you, and whether you're able to walk a line of moderation or whether abstinence is the easier path for you. You have to know what your goals are, recognize what you can and can't moderate, and, most importantly, understand how you are using food and whether you are nourishing yourself or using food in ways it wasn't meant to be used.

It's also really important to acknowledge that as your recovery evolves, your mindset may also evolve and change. Abstinence will be the answer at times in your life, while at other times, abundance might be okay. Equally, abstinence may be the answer with some foods, while there are others you might find you can be more flexible with at certain moments. Listen to your limits and be truly honest with yourself about what you can and can't handle. Be aware of changes as time passes, and recognize that this is a years-long (or even lifetime) process that is bound to adapt and alter as you adapt and alter. It's important to keep an open mind and remain flexible, knowing that what works for you in your recovery today may not work for you in your recovery tomorrow, next year, or the next decade.

Food Recovery Can Be Fun. Yes, Really!

A final thought we want to cover in this chapter on food: it's not about loss, but about gain. Many people who begin dieting feel they are losing something (remember, we did, too), but this isn't true. You are actually gaining so, so much when you put food in its proper place in life. When you approach this in the right way, food can still be fun, and recovery can be fun. We don't ever want recovery to be painful, and for us, a mark of whether the journey is successful or not is how people feel. We want you to get up every day and think, "Yes, I can do that again."

The changes you make have to be sustainable. This is something that many people fail to realize, and it's why so many diets fail. Diets are commonly viewed as temporary measures. They end, and then... you don't need us to tell you what happens.

Paige recalls a nurse she worked with in the 1990s who had seen a commercial for a new sandwich from Hardees and who proclaimed with delight that as soon as her diet was over, she was going to get one.

If you're just waiting for the diet to be over so you can jump back in the water and eat whatever you want, you're not truly in recovery. You're not making sustainable, enjoyable changes. This is why diet can not be about deprivation but about finding new ways to enjoy food so that you feel satisfied, calm, and free from cravings. Any other approach is slated for disaster and only serves to increase food obsessions and food focus.

At RFR, we want to free people from diets, from cheat days, from white-knuckling from one restrictive eating pattern to the next, and from experiencing every high and low as their eating patterns fluctuate according to arbitrary eating rules. We know that, really, all that works is making the choice to use food for nourishment (as much as possible) and stepping into a place of calm where food is in proportion with all other parts of life. So we're going to ask you now to take a few moments to think about how you use food and what roles it is serving in your life right now.

Next, in Chapter 3, we're going to start looking at the relationship between food and sleep, why sleep matters, and what people can do to make improvements here too.

CHAPTER 3

Sleep: A Successful Day In Recovery Starts The Night Before

Many people are surprised to learn that we consider sleep one of the most critical branches (if not the most critical) after food. However, good sleep is fundamental to the recovery process and to staying firmly on the lifeboat when the waves get large. Did you know that when you haven't slept enough, your body starts seeking the easiest form of energy: food?

Many of us sleep badly a lot of the time for a whole range of reasons, whether it's staying up worrying about something, working late, looking after children, trying to get on top of the domestic chores, or something else. Even without actual solid reasons, many of us find it hard to doze off, even when we're exhausted; we lie under the blankets, tossing and turning but not quite managing to slip away.

Why is sleep such a problem for so many of us in a world where we often seem to be permanently exhausted?

Before we figure that out, let's take a look at some of the impacts of poor sleep on your relationship with food. That starts with two hormones called leptin and ghrelin. Leptin is the "satiety hormone," and it reduces your desire to eat. Ghrelin is often called the "hunger hormone," and it prompts you to eat more. Sleeping too little increases the production of ghrelin and decreases the production of leptin, meaning that when you're sleep-deprived, your body is much more likely to tell you that you're hungry and you need to eat.

Furthermore, lack of sleep affects your ability to make good decisions. It reduces activity in the frontal lobe, which is responsible for impulse control and decision-making. If you're poorly rested, you lack the mental clarity to make good decisions, and you can guess where that leads. For many of us, it's a map straight to the drive-through. Added to this, your brain's reward center will be increasingly sensitive, trying to find things that will make you feel better (since nobody feels good on too little sleep). It will, therefore, seek out foods that trigger the dopamine release, and it's much harder to ignore this when you're sleep-deprived.

People are much more likely to snack - and choose unhealthy snacks to boot - when they stay up late at night. They lack impulse control, they want energy, and they're seeking rewards. The combination of all three generally leads to poor eating patterns, which can quickly become habits if you are consistently sleep-deprived.

Unfortunately, as most of us know, the modern world is not conducive to good sleep. Artificial lights and blue screens prolong our waking hours, while work and life commitments prevent us from catching up in the day. With chaotic, hectic lives and many demands on our time, a lot of us have put sleep low on the priority list, and it is our diets that suffer the effects of this (as well as our moods, physical health, and more).

This adds up to a situation where people don't have the energy to prepare good food, move their bodies, or get in touch with their spirituality. Trying to meditate when you've been up half the night with a crying toddler? It's likely to end up with you falling asleep on your mat! Everything else in life becomes difficult when you're sleeping badly, yet so many of us cut back on sleep for other commitments. We live in a strange world where prioritizing good sleep often results in you being categorized as lazy, despite how crucial sleep is for us to function!

Indeed, if you've spent any time understanding the world of addiction, you may be familiar with the HALT acronym, which we often cover at RFR. It stands for Hungry, Angry, Lonely, and Tired. It reminds people to pause (halt all activity) and check in with these feelings. These four feelings are the root cause of many of our most self-destructive behaviors, and that includes food obsession and over-eating. These feelings are a warning system that your body needs something, and you should address that before you feel worse.

If you're hungry, you might take the time to eat a nutritious snack or meal. If you're angry, you might take a breather or try some meditation. If you're lonely, you might call a friend, spend some time with your family, or plan a social night. And finally, if you're tired, you might sleep. These things may seem obvious, but it's amazing how often we fail to realize that we need to halt, check in with our bodies, and meet their needs *in appropriate ways*. That means not eating when you're actually tired or lonely but instead adequately addressing the issue so that you can feel better. Very often, when we think we need to eat, we actually just need to rest.

Although good sleep is important for everyone, we feel this is an issue that affects women in particular, and this brings us to the title of our chapter: the three Ps of sleep - premenopause, perimenopause, and postmenopause. We recognize that throughout their lives, women end up sacrificing their sleep for a whole range of reasons. We're going to explore this in more detail a little later.

The short version is that a vast number of women of all ages find themselves suffering from lack of sleep, which triggers poor eating habits, and they're totally at sea when it comes to making changes. You're one of millions if this speaks to you, and we've both been there, too.

Jamie: Self-Love and The Sleep Crypt

I recall being told that when I was a little girl, I used to rock myself to sleep. Not as some small children do, but by kneeling on my bed on all fours, placing my head against the pillow, and rocking back and forth. Sometimes, I was hitting the wall with the side of my body in an effort to get myself to drop off, to the point that my mother actually took me to a doctor because she was so concerned. What caused that? There are many possibilities, including high sugar intake, neurodivergence, and the unsettled home life, but sleep was a problem for me from the word "go," and although I've certainly had periods of better and easier sleep, it remains a big factor in my life.

I didn't have any problems during my teenage years, but when I went to college, things changed again. I think it was due to anxiety as I fought to transition my way into the adult world and struggled with the process. It left me often unable to drop off at night and constantly exhausted, day after day. I needed energy, so where did I turn? Food.

My anxiety got worse, and I became very focused on noise sensitivity. I was hyper-aware of noises around me, of a clock ticking or a fan buzzing or a phone chiming. All of these things drew my attention, and when night fell, that made it impossible to sleep. Combine that with living in a big city with lots of noise and light, and my sleep environment became impossible for me to cope with.

My food choices made it worse still. Exhausted when I got up in the morning, I went straight for the stimulant options: high calories, high sugar, high caffeine. How else was I going to get through the day? I kept eating these foods, not recognizing that they made things worse; I had no concept of "the day of and the day after" knock-on effect. I didn't realize that drinking coffee at 11 a.m. could still be keeping me awake at 11 p.m. All I knew was that the coffee got me through the first hour or two of the day, and I needed that if I wanted to survive.

Realizing that I was tired all the time, I made some early attempts to change things and improve my sleep around the time I left college. I got extra drapes and a white noise machine and found my nights were more restful. As I got older, I got ever more protective of my sleep environment. I couldn't bear even the tiniest noise in my room at night.

It got so bad that when I was in my 30s and married, my husband and I would sleep in separate rooms; he was a snorer, and I wouldn't get a wink of sleep if I lay beside him in the bed. We were both overweight, addicted to food, and loud at night. Sadly, although that setup did save me some restless nights, it exacerbated other issues and deepened our separation when problems began to occur in our marriage.

And then, what came next? Sleep apnea. It hit sometime around my early 30s. I remember waking up over and over again in the night, struggling with my own body, and then having to force myself to crawl out of bed in the morning because I was, bluntly, utterly beyond exhausted. I was moody, frustrated, upset, anxious, depressed, irritable - and every other negative emotion to be found in the book of sleep deprivation.

Sleep apnea has some serious health risks besides the mental health problems it causes. Heart disease, high blood pressure, diabetes, stroke, and more all rolled into a person who was already eating badly enough to raise those issues in other ways. I was putting myself at serious risk of permanent health problems or even death.

I found myself in a sleep study at the age of 33, and I knew I couldn't keep going like that. It coincided roughly with many of my other health problems, building up into a tidal wave of issues that left me with no choice: get out of the water or drown. I had to somehow fight my way onto the lifeboat or face being swept away to the depths of the ocean, never to be seen again.

Like my other health wake-up calls, it was the beginning of the end for my food addiction. I was too young to be that ill, to be struggling on so many counts. It was the last straw: I had to make changes if I was going to survive, both physically and mentally.

As I pulled myself, bedraggled and exhausted, onto the boat with better eating, I also focused on better sleep. I started to learn about sleep hygiene, both alongside and independently of my food recovery, and in my early 40s, I put sleep at the top of the priority list, stuck a pin in it, and forced myself to keep it there.

It was really hard at first. Many of the things that were causing me to sleep badly were things that I felt I had to do, like hitting the gym at 4 a.m., which I often did specifically because I knew it wouldn't happen later in the day, or working until late, which I did because I felt lazy otherwise.

All of those things (and many others) felt like they mattered more than getting enough hours of sleep, and I was still struggling with anxiety that made it hard to drop off at night. As I gained more tools and a better understanding of sleep, I realized that I was robbing Peter to pay Paul, and it wasn't helping anyone.

In tandem with my other recovery efforts, I began to work very hard on my sleep routine. I learned about sleep hygiene, and I began to guard my sleep hours passionately. I found that by eating better and not running my body so hard with exercise, I was able to unwind at night, drop off, and stay asleep. I began to wake up feeling more rested and less anxious. My sleep apnea eased.

I was on fire in my early 40s. Proper rest revolutionized my days and made me feel capable of anything. There were no challenges too big for me, including sticking rigorously to my diet and fueling my body with good nutrition, which in turn made it easier to sleep. Things improved a lot, but that wasn't the end of my roller coaster with sleep because my body had another surprise in store for me: perimenopause.

I want to take a moment here to point out that I'm not a doctor. Everybody experiences different symptoms as they take this journey. However, this was mine, and I know many other women have been through similar trials.

I started waking up to go to the bathroom at night. Just that disturbance was annoying, but it was quickly followed by night sweats, my first indication that perimenopause was hitting. And when your own body wakes you up every few hours feeling as though you're in an oven and you'll never be cool again, your sleep really suffers.

It was a whole new gauntlet to run, and I wasn't sure I had the energy. I'd already done my battle with sleep. I'd been there and figured out what worked. Did I have to undertake it all again?

I took up the fight. I became fastidious about my sleep hygiene practices. I went back to my blackout drapes. I told my husband that all lights must be off or covered, even tiny LEDs. Phones had to be face-down or out of the room. "The crypt," as my husband jokingly referred to our newly darkened bedroom, was essential to me if I was going to get some decent rest.

I didn't stop at the lights. Temperature got its fair share of focus, too. In fact, it's one of the few things we argue about: I must have my room in the low 70s, while my husband would rather go for mid-70s to save money. I see his point, but for me, it's about saving my health and my sanity. I need coolness to rest, and I need rest to exist.

There was another lesson I had to learn, too: respecting how much time my body needs to recuperate. My husband can get six or seven hours and wake up ready for the day. I must have eight hours. And I had to fight all the "I'm lazy" and "Do I really need it?" thoughts that cropped up whenever I saw him leap out of bed at dawn and start moving a good two hours before I was ready to emerge.

We all have those thoughts, but we have to remember that our sleep needs vary, and you *must* respect what your body tells you its quota is, especially as you get older. You can't run on half-empty; you're going to grind to a halt or burn out. Seven hours isn't enough for me, and while learning to respect that has been a slow, grudging process, I know what happens if I don't. Indeed, my sleep needs have gone up as I've aged, and I've recognized that change because I've had to.

So, what's my sleep hygiene routine these days? I've worked hard to create a habit loop for myself at night that sets me up for restful sleep. First of all, there's "the crypt," as introduced above. That's my setup, but my actions are just as important, too. That means an evening of low lights and low sounds. Sometimes, I opt for soft music or brown noise. I choose lamps with a soft glow. I avoid screens and often pick up a book (a real one, no Kindles) to ease my brain into rest. I often include stretching to counteract all the sitting that takes place in a day, and my back certainly thanks me for it!

These days, I approach sleep with a generous attitude. I let myself nap and I relish my one morning a week when I don't have to set an alarm. I doze when I can. For someone who is driven, self-disciplined, and constantly inclined to move, produce, and accomplish, it has been a rocky but immensely rewarding journey. I'm still learning to cope with the changes of perimenopause and a down-regulated thyroid, but the difference now is that I approach my sleep needs from a place of acceptance and respect rather than skepticism and self-criticism. Those did me no good.

I'd also encourage any reader who has experienced a sudden change in their sleep needs to consult with a medical professional. Sometimes, it's nothing, but sometimes, it's a sign that something is different in your body that warrants investigation. Similarly, don't ignore the change and force yourself to follow your regular routine: respect your body. Respect its needs. Respect what it tells you with exhaustion, lethargy, and a drive to grab the nearest source of sugar it can find. These things say that you need more shut-eye, and if you don't listen, you're going to get that energy elsewhere. I learned the hard way, but you don't have to.

Paige: A Sleepless Night or Two

Unlike Jamie, I've rarely suffered from sleep deprivation, and in my younger years, I made no connection between poor sleep and bad food, but when I look back, that connection shines like a beacon over some of the most sleepless nights I've had.

On April 26, 1991, at 6:45 p.m., Andover, Kansas, was struck head-on with an F5 tornado that would kill 17 people and injure 313 others. At the time, I was employed by Wesley Medical Center as an RN in the Medical Intensive Care Unit (MICU).

I was a mother with two young children, six and seven, and my husband was out of town. I'd already done a full day of parenthood and settled my children for the night, and I was pretty much ready to go to bed myself! At 9 p.m., I got the call that all hospital employees were required to report for emergency duty.

I called my mom to ask her to come and stay the night with the kids, already wondering how I was going to make it through. I was so tired, and the work hadn't even begun. I was starting an all-nighter at what should have been my bedtime, a weary mother who was already pretty much running on empty.

The initial shock of bodies lining the hallways on gurneys gave me an unexpected jolt of adrenaline as we triaged the worst cases to their respective rooms. But as the evening hours wore on and extreme fatigue took over, growing concern for how I would make it through this night plagued me. I soon became so exhausted that even the thought of driving home scared me; I'd been up for over 24 grueling hours.

It's thought that going without sleep for too long can impair your ability to drive in the same way as drinking alcohol. Being awake for at least 18 hours is the equivalent of having a blood alcohol content of 0.05%. Being awake for at least 24 hours is equal to having a blood alcohol content of 0.10%. Being the nice Mormon girl that I am, I have never been drunk, but that night, I understood what it must feel like!

To keep everyone awake, the hospital started delivering pizzas and doughnuts to all the staff. They were smart enough to know that when you are tired, the brain automatically starts seeking food as a form of energy. It's a temporary fix to what can (in normal circumstances) be solved easily by just getting some shut-eye. I remember stuffing pizza into my mouth in the early hours, desperately hoping the melty cheese and salty pepperoni would satisfy my yearning to lie down and sleep. Diet be damned, I needed something in my stomach if I was going to stay upright.

And sure, that was fine in those moments at the hospital, but that really hits the crux of the matter: diet be damned. When you need energy, your body will take it in whatever form you can get it.

That was my worst work moment, where lack of sleep was destroying my approach to food. But what about in other moments of life? Many of us think we can skimp on sleep when we're doing fun things. Who needs the brain to be rested and switched on then? But what I've found over the years is that rest matters just as much in these moments. So, let's take a few moments to talk about when I traveled to Europe, often with overnight flights, little sleep, jet lag, and, at the other end, hitting the ground running.

First of all, in Paris, where I should have known better than to head straight to the Louvre after hours on the plane. I felt like Mona Lisa was looking at me funny and I didn't care for her attitude. I have to wonder now: If first-class Paris travel was affordable, would Mona and I have hit it off better - maybe even been friends?

Jet lag is no joke. Those of you who have experienced an all-night upright flight know what I mean. It takes days to recoup from that type of sleep loss; you are operating in a drug-like state. It's that fuzzy-brained, dizzy, heavy-faced feeling you just can't shake. That level of sleep deprivation prevents you from reaching your goals. You'll never get where you want to be because the only place you want to be is taking a nap.

I stood in this incredible museum, staring up at one of the most famous paintings in the world, and I just couldn't wait for it to be over so I could find some form of comfort. I knew I should be enjoying myself, but I wasn't. What my body truly wanted was sleep, but the only thing available was food - so I took that instead. Nothing felt good, and even Mona couldn't make me smile.

What about the time when I flew to Copenhagen with a bunch of friends? One of the first things we did as we wandered, dizzy and sleepy, through the city was visit a street vendor making incredible crepes with Nutella and bananas. We had one each, and as we walked around, marveled over the city, explored and "ahhed" and touristed our way through the sites, that crepe stayed firmly fixed in my mind. I found myself thinking about it more than the beautiful history around me. I felt like I couldn't live without another one. In reality, my brain was just exhausted, and since I hadn't put sleep on my vacation menu, it was seeking any easy energy. We were in our hotel room and in our pajamas before I cracked and asked who wanted to go find that vendor and get another crepe. With exhaustion as our companion, you can guess how that ended.

Or the time I ate my way across Bruges in Belgium and gained 7 lbs. on a 5-day trip. It was like a vacation of chocolatiers, where I found myself in physical agony every time I tried to put the chocolate bag down. The only thing that would take the pain away was another bite of rich, high-pitched, homemade chocolates. Every street corner, every window display, was screaming so loudly it seemed deafening. I walked 15 hours a day to pack every experience in, and I was utterly exhausted, yet all I could think about was more chocolate.

You don't get chocolate like that in the States, which made a great excuse for gluttony. I wasn't even experiencing it: I was just shoveling it in, unconcerned with the taste, simply trying to tick the "more" box so the pain would go away. Unfortunately, it's obvious that sleep deprivation wakes the food addiction demons, and sugar in any form is easy prey. Looking back, I know that if I hadn't been out-of-my-mind exhausted, haven't-slept-in-thirty-hours tired, beside myself with weariness, I wouldn't have done that. I wouldn't have wanted my vacations to involve eating my way from one attraction to the next, but my body demanded energy, and food was the only option I gave it. Who wants to waste a trip abroad sleeping?

Well, I found out the hard way that if I didn't sleep, I really was wasting it, and in a way, that was bad for both my physical and mental health. My goal was to be there and enjoy every moment, but all I could truly think about was, "How soon until this is over?" Food eased that sensation just a little bit.

So, what have I learned after many, many lessons on the critical nature of sleep? I need it. If I don't sleep enough, I lose my ability to function and self-regulate, and I lose my sense of calm. Sleep keeps me on the lifeboat, serving as a safety line so I can reel myself back in if I do go overboard.

I now protect my sleep with every fiber of my being and schedule a minimum of a 20-minute nap every day. I call it getting ready for the second shift. Recently, I found out that 27 minutes is the right amount of time for a healthy nap without ramifications... and who am I to argue with science? All I heard was I get seven more minutes of shut-eye! I make sure I fit that nap in, even when life is crazy because I know I need it, and I know it's a key part of keeping me on track with my food.

At night, I'm equally ferocious. My sleep routine starts a couple of hours before bedtime, and I actually stop eating around 4 p.m. I'm in bed by 8:30 p.m., and yes, I do get the odd hunger twinge, but I also know I've had enough calories for the day, and if I eat at nighttime, I'm vulnerable to all those issues we discussed at the start of the chapter. I don't want to open the door of opportunity, letting the demons in, so I simply tell any hunger pains, "It's okay; I'm going to feed you again in the morning; you've had enough. Think how happy you'll be when you wake up and find you met your goals."

I know I need to wind down a couple of hours before drifting off. Washing my face and brushing my teeth are good signals to the brain that momma is tired, so it should start slowing things down. Reading or a mindless TV show happens an hour or so before I enter my darkened cavern. The fan is set to just the right speed and doubles for white noise and a cool breeze. Of course, all electronics are turned to silent, and the blackout curtains are drawn to their proper position. Another little trick is that I stop drinking several hours before bed to try to keep potty breaks to once a night.

It's hard to maintain the discipline for these things, but like Jamie, I've learned how critical it is, and I know what happens if I don't do it. Woman overboard, captain - and I don't want to go there again. Wherever I am, whatever I'm doing, I treat sleep with the same importance as my other physical needs and make sure I listen to my body's energy cues.

The RFR Takeaways

Our Sleep Needs Change as we Age

We mentioned in the introduction to this chapter that we believe sleep issues affect women more than men (you've seen the memes of the man snoring away while the woman lies awake for hours, second-guessing, worrying and thinking in a seemingly endless loop). That's definitely the case for many of us females, but there's more to it than just that; there's the hormones to consider, and the three major stages we go through - all of which affect our sleep in different ways. Let's take a look at these next.

Perimenopause is a time when women are less likely to be struggling with their sleep for physical reasons, but it's also a time when they're likely to be juggling children, careers, and chores. The three Cs that mean a good night's rest is rarely an option.

Women generally end up shouldering the brunt of caregiving for children, especially in a child's early years, when sleep may be particularly broken. This is often coupled with trying to hold down a job, keep up with domestic chores, and maintain a social life. Even if you're only balancing two Cs, you've got an awful lot on your plate and none of it is likely to be healthy!

Unfortunately, when you've got a kid in bed with you, you've been up since 3 a.m., and you've got to leave for work in 7 minutes, you're not likely to want to get up and start making a nutritious breakfast. More like grab a protein bar, throw on some clothes, and head out the door, at least for most of us. Many mothers are so busy trying to catch up that if they eat anything at all, it feels like a miracle.

Sadly, that sets up unhealthy eating habits and poor nutrition that will come back to bite you at some point, even if it's not when your children are small. When life slows down a bit (and you're looking after teenagers or empty-nesting), most of these women suddenly find that they're gaining weight as a result of physical changes in their bodies and years of bad habits around eating. It can be really hard to change this.

So, that takes us to menopause, when, for many women, restful nights become even harder to obtain. While children may be grown (and possibly gone) by this stage, natural changes within the body are likely to have an impact, and significant numbers of menopausal women suffer from sleep issues, just as Jamie has experienced. This is particularly associated with night sweats, which can seriously disturb your sleep; you're suddenly sweltering for no apparent reason, and you just have to kick the covers off or even go and stand outside just to get some relief.

Even if hot flashes don't affect you or you're not aware that your sleep has been particularly badly impacted by changes in your body, a lot of women do find that their sleep is generally less restful and more disturbed than during perimenopause. Some women develop sleep disorders, like sleep apnea, because of reductions in reproductive hormones like progesterone and estrogen. Unfortunately, many of the symptoms of sleep disorders, like feeling fatigued during the day, are also symptoms of menopause, which leads to poor diagnosis and other problems.

This is compounded by the mental health dip that many women experience as a result of menopause. Depression and anxiety may rise at this time, making it harder to fall asleep or sleep well.

These problems can continue into menopause, especially if poor sleep habits result from them. Poor sleep leaves us grumpy, emotional, frustrated, miserable, and—you guessed it—less capable of resisting ultra-processed foods.

This is often combined with a metabolism that is naturally slowing down and, for many women, a less hectic lifestyle. Think of all the pounds you shed when chasing your little one down the road or lugging buckets of laundry up and downstairs. Mothers get a real workout, often without realizing it, and if that exercise isn't replaced by something else as time passes, it often leads to serious weight gain, even for individuals who have never struggled with weight problems in the past. All of these issues come together, tilting the lifeboat at a dramatic angle and making it much harder for us to stay on board.

Making Sleep Hygiene Work For You

There aren't any magic bullets when it comes to sleep, and we want to caveat our advice in this chapter by saying that you may wish to consult with your healthcare professional if you're suffering from sleep disruptions or if you're concerned about sleep disorders. Some issues require medical intervention. However, there are often things that you can do at home to improve your sleep, following a concept known as sleep hygiene. It's not about showering before you go to bed; it's about implementing habits that are conducive to easy, restful, high-quality sleep.

Take a bit of time to assess your "habit loop" and how you prepare your body for sleep. Are you setting yourself up for success or for failure? Watching TV (especially stimulating, high-action shows), using social media, or gaming before bed can all make it harder to drop off because they engage your brain and often increase the adrenaline in your system. Exploring what kind of habit loop you're creating before you go to sleep can help you identify areas where improvement may be needed. Are you setting yourself up for success or failure when you finally close your eyes?

Sleep hygiene often involves multiple areas, with one of the most important being the creation of an ideal sleep environment. Your bedroom should be dark, relaxing, quiet, and set to a comfortable temperature. That might mean purchasing blackout curtains, installing a fan, or investing in more comfortable bedding and sleepwear. A cool room tends to be better for sleep than a hot one, but find a temperature that feels right to you.

It should also entail removing all electronic devices from the bedroom. No TVs, computers, or smartphones. If you need sound to fall asleep, consider a radio or another device that doesn't emit light, or silence all notifications and other sounds before putting your smartphone in your room. We know that blue light keeps us up later, so avoid using screens before bed and install programs to reduce the blue light (most devices now have blue light filters).

It's also a good idea to implement consistency in your habits as much as possible. Going to bed and getting up at approximately the same time every day will help regulate your circadian rhythm, making it easier for you to fall asleep quickly and wake up effectively. We recommend an early-to-bed, early-to-rise regimen (while recognizing that this doesn't work for everyone) because decision fatigue often kicks in during the evening hours, and this can leave you vulnerable to unhealthy snacking.

Tied in with this, it's important to avoid eating a large meal at the end of the day. Large meals will often keep your body active, trying to digest the food, which can reduce your overall sleep quality and make you restless and uncomfortable. It takes several hours to digest food, so the disruption can be significant and could also lead to issues like acid reflux.

Alcohol should similarly be avoided before bed; while you might feel as though a drink or two helps you unwind and promotes a sense of sleepiness, it's not helpful to restful sleep. It will often wake you up after just a few hours and leave you feeling restless and unable to doze off again.

We're going to look at exercise more fully in the next chapter, but it's also key to good sleep. However, when it comes to physical activity, timing matters. Don't undertake a big workout just before bed! If you get your heart rate up and your adrenaline pumping and then lie down to sleep... well, we can all see that isn't going to go well. Instead, try to fit your exercise in much earlier in the day so your body has time to come down from it and relax again.

It's also important not to make sleep a source of stress. If it's not coming naturally, you shouldn't get all worked up and worried; that's a sure way to postpone sleep even further. Instead, if you're not sleeping, it's best to get up and sit somewhere comfortable with a book or some other relaxing activity. You will hopefully find that sleep gradually washes over you, and you are then ready to go back to bed and try again.

Some people find that other techniques, such as meditating before bed, journaling, making a to-do list for the next day, or listening to soothing music, can help. Try various methods and see what works for you, but ultimately, prioritize good sleep and seek help if you find that you're struggling with it.

Next, we want to come back to the question we asked at the start of the chapter: Why is sleep such a problem for so many of us in a world where we often seem to be permanently exhausted? We've given many reasons for that now, most of which boil down to hectic lives and hormones, poor mental health, bad diets, etc., but now we want to present another key reason many people don't sleep well: we don't prioritize it.

That thought might make some of us feel defensive because it seems like a criticism, but it's not. Instead, it's a recognition that many of us let other things in life become more important than sleep for a whole range of - sometimes very good - reasons. Sometimes, there's no avoiding it: sleep takes a backseat, and there's nothing we can do. Emergency tornadoes, small children, family illnesses, or just a particularly hectic week at work - we've all been there, and we have to recognize that it's okay for it to happen occasionally.

However, when sleep is constantly taking a backseat, and you're never finding it at the top of the agenda, it's time for a wake-up call (no pun intended). You're not doing your eating habits or the rest of your physical health and mental well-being any favors if you consistently don't get enough sleep.

The answer is almost always that something else has to give way. It may be that you sacrifice your 20-minute tidy-up while the toddler's napping and instead take a nap yourself. It might be saying "no" to a social Saturday and catching up on chores so you can be better rested throughout the week. It might be ordering groceries online to save yourself shopping time, getting a cleaner once a week, asking your partner to step up with the childcare, taking a day off work to recharge, or a myriad of other things.

Only you can judge what it's practical to say "no" to, how to adjust your schedule, and what you can and can't do, but take this as a sign to start putting sleep higher on the agenda and looking for ways to get your shut-eye. Bring your bedtime forward an hour, be disciplined, and remind yourself of all the health benefits that come with sleeping well. Your body matters enough to give it sufficient sleep; don't forget this! Even the important stuff in life shouldn't take priority over your health all the time, and your sleep is, to an extent, your health.

You're likely to find that when you prioritize sleep and good sleep hygiene, at least some of the time, you have better control over your eating habits. And the great thing about this is that the rest of your branches of recovery will grow!

Sleep isn't the second-most important branch for everyone, but it's very key to staying on the lifeboat of recovery.

Next, we're going to look at movement, another of our major branches - and don't worry; we're not just going to tell you to get to the gym.

CHAPTER 4

The Magic Of Movement

I t's going to surprise no one that movement is one of our core branches, one of the biggest factors in recovery and in taking care of your body. It's also a branch that so many people we see struggle with for so many different reasons. Exercising, especially in the early days, is really tough. It takes a lot of discipline, motivation, and drive to start exercising regularly, and if you're thinking, "I just don't want to," you're a very long way from alone.

We have both been in the "don't want to" or "can't do it" categories, and we understand that feeling immensely. If exercise feels like a huge block in your journey to recovery, that's okay; we're going to give you strategies that will reduce that feeling and give you ways through. However, like the other main branches, there's not really any room for compromise here: movement is part of health, both physical and mental, and you need to be moving if you want to stay on that lifeboat and keep yourself healthy and happy.

More and more people are becoming aware of how critical movement is for both physical and mental health. We know we need to move and keep ourselves fit, but actually doing it is a serious challenge for most of us, from all phases of life and in all situations. Neither of us began our lives as keen athletes nor spent many of our years doing triathlons, competing in marathons, or training for the Olympics. Nonetheless, movement has generated magic for both of us, and that magic is an inherent part of getting better.

Some people think that movement has to involve something highly physical and strenuous. They picture the typical muscular gym buff, dripping with sweat as they lift dumbells the size of dinner plates... and no wonder they get scared off. If you don't go, the gym can feel like an unwelcoming trial by fire, where everybody will laugh at your efforts and call you names behind your back.

That's the block that many people run into when they consider movement: they assume that it must be at the gym, that it must be intense, and that it must be unpleasant and grueling to be sufficiently rewarding. Fortunately, none of that is true, and if you can release those assumptions and move forward, you'll find that exercise becomes a key plank in the raft keeping you out of the water - not an extra chore that is trying to push you under.

But why should you exercise? Well, we're going to be brief here because there are so many advantages, and you're probably familiar with most of them already. Here are our top reasons for exercising:

- To increase your bone density, protecting yourself from falls and making your body stronger
- To prevent weight gain and maintain a healthy weight. Even a small amount of exercise will give your metabolism a good boost and help you shed extra weight
- To increase your muscle mass, making it easier to maintain your strength. Remember that muscles and bones tend to weaken when we age, but exercise can help maintain them
- To reduce the risk of weight-related diseases, including high blood pressure, diabetes, cardiovascular issues, cholesterol, etc.
- To create a meditative-like state where you are focused on your body and its movements; this builds a sense of connection with who you are and the power you control, making you feel more in tune with your body and potentially helping you make healthier food choices
- To provide a mood boost by releasing endorphins into the bloodstream and creating a sense of accomplishment and motivation
- To improve your sleep. Exercise helps us to enjoy better, longer sleep because it uses up energy, tires us out, and makes it easier to relax at the end of the day[1]
- To connect with others. Not everybody wants to exercise with those around them, but there's a wonderful social scene that you can tap into if you want to

---

[1] Alnawwar, M. A., Alraddadi, M. I., Algethmi, R. A., Salem, G. A., Salem, M., & Alharbi, A. A. (2023). The effect of physical activity on sleep quality and sleep disorder: A systematic review. *Cureus*. https://doi.org/10.7759/cureus.43595

- To maintain balance, which often worsens as we age, and to reduce the risk of falls and injuries
- To improve brain health. It's thought that regularly exercising increases the blood flow to the brain, which could potentially help protect mental functioning and improve your ability to focus, even as you age

That's not an exhaustive list, but it gives you some idea of just how extensive the benefits of exercising can be. Movement really is magic... but for a lot of us, it feels intimidating. Getting started is often a marathon journey just by itself. With that in mind, let's take a look at our exercise journeys and then begin exploring how you can make exercise a key element of your recovery journey.

Jamie: Movement Is So Much More Than Just Physical

When I started my recovery journey, movement was like a dirty word. I did not want to do it, and I did not know how to do it. Honestly, I couldn't have done it healthily because I was so big. It was both painful and taxing, just moving my body from A to B. I used to get tired simply from walking fast or even standing up and speaking for long periods. It was enormously stressful for me, both physically and emotionally. I had no idea how I'd go about starting my journey with movement, and for a while, it wasn't on the agenda anyway.

Instead, I worked with my dietician and my counselor to get my food in order and bring down my weight. We talked about creating healthy portions of food and which foods to choose and avoid, not how to exercise my body. Essentially, they wanted to pull me back from the cliff edge before they helped me with any other elements of health, so in the early parts of my journey, movement wasn't a factor - at least as far as I knew.

However, I was actually already doing quite a lot of moving just in terms of managing my own body, so I had a fair bit of muscle tone and reasonable cardiovascular fitness even when I began, simply because I had to put so much effort into moving myself. When I began eating right, I quickly started to drop the pounds and with that came a change: energy. I wasn't spending it on moving my body and suddenly, I had it to spare. It was a new feeling.

Instead of being exhausted simply from the effort of moving myself, I began to find that I wanted to move. I had excess energy that I was anxious to burn off. When I started walking, it wasn't because I particularly wanted to walk or because I thought it would help me lose weight; it was simply that since I was carrying less weight, I had energy left over, and I had to burn it off in some way. I began to walk regularly, and to my surprise, I found that people were enormously kind and encouraging toward me.

I would listen to audiobooks and music as I walked, and later, as I got fitter, I began taking calls while moving. I no longer got out of breath. I felt good. Moving felt good, and that was such a revelation to me. It was still a gradual process and I was taking it slowly, but what a difference I saw.

The following summer, I got myself a bike. It was a tricky decision because I wasn't all that comfortable with bikes. I was still heavy, I didn't have great balance, and I was afraid that if I fell off, I might injure myself. I did have to be careful, but pretty much as soon as I got on a bike, I realized... Wow, I love this.

The fear went (for the most part), and I started to gain confidence. I enjoyed the bike's freedom, speed, power and energy. I quickly gained the muscles to cycle, and I felt really good. Soon, I was able to cycle faster and more often, and my body began changing even more quickly. I could have spent hours on my bike; I loved it that much.

Unfortunately, winter in Wisconsin wasn't friendly to cyclists, and when the colder weather came, I realized I'd have to find another option for burning off my extra energy; I couldn't bike safely on the icy roads. That's where the gym entered my life, though without any enthusiasm on my part.

I was not comfortable in the gym. In the early days, I would go in, use the treadmill or an elliptical trainer for 30 minutes, and then leave as quickly as I could. I wanted to get out of those doors as soon as possible. I didn't set foot in any other areas. I didn't talk to anyone, explore any of the other equipment, use the weights, or anything else; I just did my thing and left. For a while, that was my gym experience - pretty solitary.

Indeed, I treated the gym almost like a punishment at times. I'd got myself into this mess, and now I had to pay for it by putting myself through this uncomfortable experience every day. "Your own fault," I would tell myself whenever I had thoughts about not wanting to go, about possibly skipping a session. I faced a lot of internal shame and self-judgment, and at points, it was very hard for me to keep going, even though I knew that if I could get past that lack of confidence, I'd have something of value. It was a struggle just to step into the building a lot of the time, even though the only negativity came from me.

Gradually, though, I became more comfortable in the space and to feel curious about the other machines. As my confidence grew, I tried a few out, and as people in the gym began to recognize me as a regular, they'd talk to me, offer me advice, and invite me to try things. They were kind and warm and welcoming; far from the stereotype.

That's how I ended up in my first spin class. That was fabulous. Suddenly, I could enjoy my love of cycling indoors, and I was at it every day. Twelve years later, I still love my stationary bike, which has no chance of tipping me off and no real risk of injury - where I can go as fast as I want and cycle for as long as I like. It's perfect.

My body wasn't the only thing being reshaped by my better diet and hours in the gym, though. As my looks changed, so too did my confidence. I started to feel acceptable in the exercise space and began attending more classes. I remember thinking, "What am I doing? I'm so uncoordinated, and I've no idea how to move," but those thoughts only came from me. Outwardly, everyone was very kind; I never heard a negative comment from anyone while I was there.

I soon became part of a truly beautiful community in the gym there. These were people I never would have interacted with before, people who were very fit and active, very lively, very social - and truly wonderful in a whole myriad of ways. Soon, my gym became my support network and social outlet, a place where I loved to be. I could and did spend hours in the gym, and a place that had once been so uncomfortable became like a second home - a home I loved.

I met personal trainers and class instructors and began hanging out with them. The atmosphere was amazing. Everyone wanted everybody else to do well, celebrated each other, and encouraged each other. You could ask anybody for help, and they'd be there, doing their best to guide you toward your next goal.

After about four or five years, I decided to compete in body-building/fitness competitions, partly to see if I could get to the stage. I began intensive training, talking with fitness instructors and attending group training sessions. In between, I ran, did cardio, lifted weights, and participated in 5Ks and other competitions. By this point, I'd lost a lot of weight and was reshaping my body in ways that felt immensely rewarding.

I didn't want to do it forever, and indeed, I think I almost wanted to prove to myself that I could work my way back out of the restriction that it took to get to the stage. Many people in the body-building world get sucked in so deeply they can't pull themselves back from it. In a way, it was like testing my ability to withstand another form of addiction. I did it for a time, learned a lot, and then left it behind.

I gained so much from those times, and I still deeply love the community I found through the activity. Overall, it was a wonderful experience, both mentally and physically, giving me a totally different mindset and a different approach to the challenges I faced in life. It gave me resilience and strength and a sense of self that has stayed with me to this day. Empowering my physical body empowered all areas of my life with strength and has served me since.

When I got divorced and had to leave the area, it was a horrible, dark time for me. Even though I had to leave that community and the people I loved behind, I was still deeply grateful for the mental resilience and fortitude they had taught me. That has lasted across moves, across years, across other friendships, and it has helped me channel my emotions into my fitness.

My fitness mindset has helped me between counseling sessions, at work, and through dark periods. In the hardest parts of my life, I would just get up and move. It got me out of bed and gave me a feeling of control, even when there wasn't much I could control for the rest of my life, especially during my divorce. Fitness let me put other difficulties aside for a while so I could just move my body. In some ways, it's a form of meditation where everything else melts away, and I can just focus on myself. In other ways, I used it as a means of processing anger and sadness. Nothing moves out feelings of fury like slamming a medicine ball on the ground ten times every five minutes.

In 2020, when the pandemic forced everything to close - including my gym at the time - I lost my social outlet and physical connection in one day. It was a huge blow. I went from a group mindset and morning gym routine to exercising by myself in an apartment with no equipment and no ability to connect with the outside world. I knew that the statistics were not in my favor if I got the virus, so I couldn't afford to let my fitness slip at this time. I also knew that, being shut in my house and unable to go anywhere or do anything, my fitness was the only thing keeping me from losing my mind. I had no choice but to exercise.

At this point, I was alone, single, and very unsure of the future, but I was determined to stay on the lifeboat and keep going. I bought a spin bike from Amazon. I remember opening it and seeing the "2 people assembly required" paperwork, but I had just me, alone in my home, and I was going to get that bike up if it killed me.

I had never put anything together in my life. I sat, looking at the pieces, and I thought to myself, "Alright, here we go." It was another challenge, another opportunity to succeed. The marked difference in my approach to it still astonishes me. I didn't want to run away or find an excuse or avoid it. Yes, this would be hard, but I was capable, and I was going to do it.

And after a few hours, I had my bike assembled. My first ride on that bike felt phenomenal. I kept going and going, feeling the thrill of exercising, the exhilaration of having put the bike together myself, and the sudden rush of realization that I didn't have to lose my fitness just because my gym was gone. It was like the floor was back under my feet suddenly. I was going to be okay. I couldn't believe I had achieved it, but I had. Fitness had taught me the important life lesson of moving through the pain and discomfort to find the rewards on the other side.

I fell in love with having my own gym at home, a space where I could work out whenever I needed to. I soon had more equipment and gave up on the public gym. Certainly, I missed the community, but the flexibility and accessibility of the equipment at home were worth it, and the gym mindset stayed with me nonetheless.

I've carried that with me to this day, and even now, it helps me immensely when times are challenging. I found that often, fitness was for my mind as much as my body. Fitness let me find a beautiful place where I could come into my own in my body, love the sense of power and strength, and feel good about myself.

I was not someone who had ever seen myself taking up a gym membership. Remember, I was morbidly obese, at around 400 lbs. I nearly killed myself with food. All I did to get there was start walking because I felt restless, and that was the catalyst, the push. You don't have to go as far as I did to succeed, either. Just walking or whatever other form of exercise appeals to you can be enough. Movement, in all its forms, is key to recovering and finding the strength and beauty in your body.

Ultimately, exercise gave me another avenue for letting in peace and self-love, another means of changing how I felt about my body. Movement became like magic, reminding me that my body was strong, powerful, and worthy of care. Without movement, I don't think I would have found that level of connection and sense of strength, even if I had lost weight through dieting. Movement made me proud of my body, not just for how it looked but for how strong it was and for how much power lay within me. It made me comfortable in my own skin and gave me a sense of connection with myself.

Many people who use food for comfort feel alienated from their bodies and out of control of how they handle them. Turning to movement changes that. It's another avenue for finding connection, focus, balance, and a sense of calm. For me, it was an unexpected benefit, but I know that exercise will be with me for the rest of my life, and it is invaluable—both for my recovery and simply for my sense of self.

Paige: When Your Body Moves, Your Brain Grooves

I want to start my story by saying that, in some ways, I've always been an exercise junkie. Climbing everything I could get a toehold on from my earliest memory, which I'm sure my parents loved. Perhaps because of my proclivity for sugar, I had a lot of movement in me from sun up to sun down, and I used it. However, as I've aged, I don't take exercise for granted, as just a standard part of my life. I know how much I need it! Most weeks, I exercise 6 days out of 7 (okay, it's usually 7 out of 7 with light days built in). I have to do this for my mental release because otherwise, I get wound very tight. I find that I can either take nervous pills or put on a pair of tennis shoes, so sneakers it is.

Exercise settles and calms me. I like to think of it as active meditation. It helps me think things through; I am constantly processing while I'm exercising. And I can, in seconds, count the benefits of exercise: I'm a nicer person, I sleep better, I have more energy, and I'm not as anxious about life, especially food. Exercise gives me that sense of control and power, reveals a source of structure, and massively increases the chances of me hitting other goals. It also helps me control my calories and weight. It's a safety net against getting sick, giving me a higher baseline so I can bounce back faster if illness does strike.

I would be remiss if I didn't mention the mental health benefits we can glean from exercise; this is one of the biggest draws for me. Sure, I love the calorie burn and feeling like a "badass" when I leave the gym, but it's really those friendly little endorphins that get me through the day. Nothing can replace those uppers.

However, I don't want you to read this and feel like exercise is easy for me, that I'm one of those lucky few who just loves going to the gym. While I have to move to keep myself healthy both mentally and physically, it doesn't mean I always feel like moving.

I wake up at 5 a.m. Do I want to drag myself upright and go challenge my body? Honestly, no. I don't. There are many days when I would rather stay under the blankets and hit "snooze," especially in the winter. It's cold outside, I'm still tired, and it's still dark. It's a real struggle to get up. We've all felt this - the bargaining, the desire to just stay put, the longing to snuggle back into the cocoon, the white lie of "later"... (we all know how this ends). But the reality is, if I only do what feels good in the moment, I would never get up, and growth would become a negative concept.

And this is where discipline comes in more than motivation, or as I like to say, discipline trumps motivation every time. Motivation is great, but it can only take you so far. I depend on discipline to get myself up. I know that pretty much every person on the planet wants to stay in bed; it's natural because we are wired for comfort, but I owe it to my body to get up and take care of business. Goals are much harder to reach horizontally.

When it seems impossible to drag yourself out of the sheets and hit the ground running, those are the moments that matter the most. When desire whispers to just curl up, hug the pillow, and slip away again... don't listen. Get up, get out of bed, and get moving. It will be over very soon, and you'll have set yourself up for a day of success. You'll have accomplished one of the big tasks on your to-do list, and that's a far better feeling than giving in to the warm blankets, believe me (and daydreaming of my nap later doesn't hurt). We do what we do for how we feel after.

What really speaks to my brain when all I want to do is pull up the blankets and doze off again, is the understanding that this is where I harness my true sense of power. Being willing to do something that I don't want to do because I'm looking at long-term results, not short-term gratification, is an amazing feeling. I know, as well as every other person, that exercising is hard. I also know that a sedentary lifestyle is harder in the long term. #adulting

And here's a curious thing I found about movement: when you muster the strength to overcome physical challenges, you increase your ability to take on mental challenges. It's like the strength in your muscles translates to the strength in your mind. Move a muscle, move a thought. A strange idea, but I remember an occasion in 2012 when my husband was facing a bone marrow transplant, and I was terrified at the prospect. I decided to climb Pikes Peak for the first time with my youngest daughter, and as I endured 13 uphill miles, the only phrase I allowed into my head was, "If I can do this, I can do anything."

When we reached the top, I cried (full disclosure, sobbed like a baby ... it might have been the altitude), and I've been climbing mountains ever since. There's nothing like a mountain to sweep away your woes and make you feel invincible. There's nothing like training your body to increase your sense of self and tap into your greatest capabilities.

In some ways, I think recovery has less to do with the right food plan and more to do with filling your life with meaning in as many ways as possible, thus organically assigning food to its natural position and priority. A necessity, and at times enjoyable, but not an all-consuming presence. I find that if I get my thrills and endorphins from moving my body, connecting with others, and accomplishing my goals, food shifts into its proper position, becoming a catalyst that helps us live and reach goals rather than encouraging us to simply live to eat.

That's why movement is so key to our 16 branches of recovery. It helps with balance. It helps with peace, calmness, and satisfaction. It provides that lovely, gentle dopamine drip that satisfies your brain. Without it, the addicted brain has one desire: "more," and it won't stop seeking it. Making a pre-emptive strike in recovery can be a vital strategic move in keeping the brain chatter to a minimum.

I also want to stress something about taking it slowly. I remember when I decided I wanted to be a runner. When I began, I didn't start by running a half-marathon all at once. I started by running a minute, walking a minute, running, walking, gradually building up my muscles and my endurance. One of my biggest accomplishments ever was when I ran my first mile without stopping.

Interestingly, it took about six weeks of training to run that first 5280 ft without taking a break, which ironically was the same period it took for me to train for a half-marathon once I was a consistent runner. The same amount of time to train for one mile as to train for a half-marathon!

Those early days took so much effort and patience before I started seeing results, but it was worth it. I just had to stay focused on the goal. I'm not exaggerating when I say that I got as much euphoria and pride from my first mile as my first half-marathon. In that first mile lay hours of endurance, sweating, exhaustion, and "I don't want to." When I succeeded, I had proven to myself that I had the drive, ambition, and ability to meet my goals. I wanted to succeed in that mile more than I wanted to sit down or stay in bed.

These types of accomplishments can then parlay into other areas of our lives. I knew I could face challenges head-on. My mantra is, "Alexanders do hard things." So, when it came to my sugar detox, I knew what I was made of. I knew I could go the distance, and those first six weeks were hard, but I had a training program for that, too. After those first six weeks, I had developed habits that were solidly in place, keeping me safe. Never limit yourself; you don't know what you are capable of until you try! It starts with desire, and my initial desire was to make it through those first crucial six days, which are the most critical in making it through those first six weeks. The good news is that it gets easier after that.

Speaking of progress, once you have built a foundation, you can use that as a springboard for other, more exciting goals. When it comes to exercise, the places it can take you if you're dedicated are truly amazing. For example, I didn't start out climbing the Grand Canyon, and I know not everyone will go there, but I've been twice, and both times were incredible experiences in their different ways.

On April 20th, 2024, I did a "redo" of my first Grand Canyon experience (which was something of a disaster, involving a 4-day hike with a 30-lb. poorly fitted backpack and bad shoes). My redo was a pinnacle of my lifetime's dedication to movement and an experience like no other.

At 6:12 a.m., seven other fanatics and I set out at the South Kaibab Trailhead and walked downhill for four hours. We dropped about a mile in elevation and covered seven miles of switchbacks (zigzags) as we headed for the Colorado River.

While dodging potholes and little piles of poo left by the caravan of mules, the question of how movement supports recovery percolated in my mind. The morning was filled with deep thoughts and purposeful steps, all the while soaking in the Canyon's beauty, that ominous, colorful hole in the earth. This felt like a great challenge, a momentous landscape with hot sun and sore feet... and I was determined that this time, I wouldn't be beaten by it. Soon, though, I realized that as difficult as it was, it was nothing compared with the fight of giving up sugar.

You may already be familiar with the idea that the greater the challenge, the greater the reward. It might sound silly, but one of the hardest things I have ever done was giving up sugar. Nothing else has tested my limits to that extreme. Nothing else has called on every fiber of my being with such force. Nothing else has left me feeling as desperate, as incapable of rising to the occasion... and as good when I was successful. Yes, I loved sugar that much, and no, I am not exaggerating.

As I continued to cover the dusty trail of the Canyon, I kept repeating one of my mother's sayings in my head: "This too shall pass." I knew that the difficulties of the Canyon, tough and exhausting though the trail was, wouldn't last forever, just as my cravings for sugar couldn't last forever. They were both testing grounds to determine what I was made of. It's this mindset that gets me through all my exercise, hard or easy, long or short.

There was another truth that the Canyon gifted me as we paused for a desperately needed break at the bottom. I sat with my feet dangling in the river, soothing the blisters forming on the undersides of my toes. The friction of walking downhill creates havoc on a fresh pedicure. As my tootsies cooled and my overtaxed joints and ligaments took a break, it occurred to me how important it is to stay on the path that provides direction.

Regardless of your goal, never giving up is the greatest ally you can have, followed shortly by having a structure and a plan. Once you have a plan, you have direction and know where to start, and that's what opens the door to progress. Remember, too, that one step in the right direction is still one step in the right direction; don't ever minimize success.

We were a long way from done at this point, of course. I had almost 12 hours that day to muse over movement and think about recovery, and perhaps most importantly, to appreciate all the things my body could do because of the time

I had put into training it. The thousands of mornings of rising early (thanks to early nights) and moving my body, and every grateful moment of "I don't want to, but I'm going to anyway." These woven fibers knitted themselves together and carried me to the finish line as the sun began to set in the Arizona sky.

We finished our day at 5:54 p.m., summiting the Bright Angel Trail. Looking back at our reward, the breathtaking vista of the Canyon, I knew it had paid off and would continue to pay off in the following days. The real bonus would lie in the sore muscles and aches, the proof that I had conquered.

I was exhausted but elated, thrilled with my own accomplishments and my efforts. I could see that practicing movement lets our bodies pay us back in so many ways, especially in letting us recoup to baseline more quickly. The same is true of food addiction recovery. When we consistently apply our efforts to honing our recovery skills, we have a better ability to take care of ourselves when challenges arise... and they will arise. That's when we can draw from the well of experience, practice, and commitment.

The last thing I will say about movement is that I can't say enough about movement. I ran for 30 years until my old lady hips and knees told me I needed a new adrenaline rush, and that's when I turned to mountain climbing and weight lifting. So long half-marathons, hello dumbells and hiking sticks. My point is keep moving. Whatever that looks like, fits into your schedule wherever you are. Just do something. Our bodies were designed to move, not sit, and movement is a critical component. We need all the natural good ju-ju we can get when rewiring those addicted snow-blown tracks in our brains, and putting one foot in front of the other is a great place to start!

The RFR Takeaways

How Do You Overcome The Exercise Hurdle?

In both of our stories, you've hopefully seen that we faced our own challenges with getting into movement, but our challenges aren't going to be the same as yours. That's why we now want to spend a bit of time looking at the most common problems that stop people from exercising and how you can start resolving those. Let's break these down and work with them.

I don't have time to exercise.

This is probably the most common trap that people fall into, and it probably feels very true for a lot of people. We are already so busy that how can you possibly also fit an hour of exercise in every single day when you're barely managing to keep up with household chores, manage children, juggle social commitments, cook, etc.?

There are several answers to this. The first is that you should drop that mentality (even if it's somewhat true) because it won't help you. If you think you never have time to exercise, you're creating a self-fulfilling prophecy that makes it a lot harder to even try. Not a good way to start!

Next, look at your day. As we mentioned above, we both exercise first thing because this is what helps us make space for it (and it has a lot of other benefits, too). Can you shift both your bedtime and your wake time forward by an hour (or even half an hour) to give yourself more time in the morning? Lay out your clothes? Prep your breakfast in advance?

Making your morning run smoothly will give you a better chance of exercising first thing. However, it's not feasible for everyone, so don't feel you have to exercise first thing. If this doesn't work for you, consider other slots in your day. How about a walk at lunchtime? Half an hour at the gym when you leave work? Cycling home?

There are many ways to make exercise part of your daily routine and incorporate it into things you are already doing. Look for a slot of time that you could repurpose or make multipurpose, and try to fit in at least a little bit of exercise. You'll soon find yourself keen to do more. It also really helps to choose an activity you enjoy at least a bit, so this doesn't feel like such a chore. There are many exercise options out there; look through them and find one you love.

Think of this in another way. When you say you don't have time to exercise, you are sending a subliminal message to your body that it isn't worth 20 minutes to an hour each day. That's all it takes to increase your fitness and make you healthier, and your body is worth that. Remember that when you invest in self-care, which includes good food, good sleep, and good movement, you tell your body that it matters, and you increase your self-esteem.

Here, of course, we want to take a moment to acknowledge you if you feel it's hard to fit the gym (or any kind of exercise) into your day. It is hard! We all lead busy lives, working long hours and struggling against the constant pull of demands on our time. However, if you're really dedicated to it, you'll find that you make time because it feels good! Whether it means pulling your morning alarm (and your bedtime) forward to give yourself an extra hour in the mornings or ditching social media to bump up your free hours, it can be done.

It's not comfortable. Or, I'm afraid of hurting myself.

This is a common fear, especially for people who struggle with food addiction, and it's also a very valid point. You don't want to hurt yourself. That's why it's important to ease into exercise smoothly and gently, giving your body time to adjust. While a good workout certainly can be uncomfortable, you don't have to get there straight away, and you don't have to push your body to its limits.

Instead, ease in. Start by walking, doing five minutes of squats, or ten minutes of Pilates. Try some yoga. Go gently on your body, and don't think that exercise has to be grueling to be rewarding. If you're moving your body, you're working magic, no matter what. Remember to listen to what your muscles are telling you, and don't go beyond your limits.

I can't afford to go to the gym. I'm afraid people will judge me.

You don't have to go to the gym. Exercise happens all over the place, not just in dedicated buildings. You can exercise outside or turn on YouTube and exercise in your bedroom. You can exercise anywhere you feel comfortable. You could take up hiking if you live in a good area, go for swims, or simply stroll briskly around the block.

Of course, a gym membership is great for some people, and it offers some amazing benefits in terms of community. Once the nerves of being in an unfamiliar space pass, gyms are often very welcoming and inclusive places, but you don't have to go if you don't want to (and remember, you can always try it later if you find yourself more at ease with the idea somewhere down the line).

I don't think I'd enjoy working out.

This is another common misconception. Actually, working out makes you feel good. Remember, it releases endorphins that make you feel good and help reduce stress, so it's a really proactive way to elevate your mood. Most of us don't feel like working out when our moods are low, or we're stressed, but it's one of the best ways to kick the bad mood aside and make yourself feel better.

One of the amazing things about exercise is that it gives you a great sense of power, even if you're not in control in every area of your life. You can massively increase your mental health by reminding yourself what your body can do.

Both of us find that exercise makes us more relaxed and that the sense of accomplishment after a workout session is incomparable with other feelings. You can give yourself such a sense of freshness and vitality just by getting your heart pumping. You also remind your body that you care about it, and you want to acknowledge its efforts by keeping it in good shape - and that's really good for your sense of self-esteem. All in all, this is a myth you've got to put aside. Until you've actually tried (consistently) working out and found that it makes you miserable, you simply don't know - and those who do exercise will tell you how much they love it.

One of our key tips here is to look for movement you can enjoy and find ways to make exercise fun. If there's an exercise that you want to do but you don't enjoy, why not get together with a group of friends while you do it? You can find a lot of comfort and relief in being able to chat while you do something hard, and at the end of a session like this, you'll feel on top of the world, both from the social boost and from the success and knowledge that the session is over!

Bear in mind that there are theories that we are most like the five people closest to us. Hanging out with high achievers means you get pulled along in the draft. Most high achievers, unsurprisingly, are also exercisers. They view obstacles not as impediments but as opportunities for learning and development. This is often referred to as a growth mindset, and it empowers you to embrace challenges with enthusiasm and resilience.

I don't want to work out every day.

Remember that exercise is flexible: you don't have to! If some days are really tough for you, you don't have to build exercise into your everyday routine or feel like you must commit 100% from now until the day you die to never take a break. That said, habit and commitment are key to exercise, and you can't schedule a "rest day" 7 days a week!

You should, therefore, build an exercise routine that feels right for you. Even if you start by only committing to exercising one day a week or three days a week, you'll be doing more than you are now. You can then build up to whatever feels sustainable. Don't think about the long-term here; focus on the now, on moving your body in a way that feels good. Once you persuade your brain that you like exercise, you might feel pretty differently about that "every day."

That isn't to say that exercise is easy for those who do it every day. It requires a lot of discipline. However, remember that it is just a relatively short portion of your day; once you've done your twenty minutes, half hour, hour, or whatever, it's over, and you can move on.

Both of us have days when we don't want to work out. We don't always want to exercise, but it's part of general body maintenance. You may also find that mood follows action. Don't wait until you feel like working out; just start. From there, the endorphins will kick in and (hopefully!) the sense of accomplishment will give you the boost needed to finish.

Often, you'll find that if you just start, it's not nearly as hard as you thought it would be. Many of us build exercising up into a big deal in our heads because we think it's going to be hot and hard and unpleasant. The reality is, it doesn't have to be, and even if it is, it will be over pretty quickly, leaving you feeling full of power and control. In fact, some of the exercise sessions that you least want to do end up being the most rewarding because at the end of them, you can admire yourself for your discipline and motivation, getting a strong sense of accomplishment.

I'm too stressed out right now.

Many people feel like adding exercise to their list of tasks in a day will increase their stress, but it's really the opposite. Because exercise releases endorphins and makes you feel less stressed, including it in your daily routine is often a great way to combat stress.

Exercise also gives you a break from stress. It involves taking a bit of time out from whatever is going on in your life to focus on your body. Similar to meditation, this provides a space in which your mind can pay attention to something else. Exercise often brings you a sense of calm. It helps you put the source of stress into perspective rather than allowing it to be an all-consuming presence in your life.

We're not saying here that you've failed if you sometimes have to take a break from exercise to focus on the biggest challenges in life; it's okay to listen to your body if it wants self-care in other forms, such as more sleep, relaxation, etc. However, for the most part, exercise will rejuvenate and refresh you, helping you feel more balanced. Remember, too, that the sense of power it gives you will often help you feel more in control of the difficult situation, even if it makes no tangible difference. It works!

I don't think I will stay motivated.

Here, you're potentially falling into that trap of sabotaging yourself before you start something because you're afraid you'll feel more disappointed if you start it and then give up. Better not to exercise at all, right?

No, and you know it. We can't afford to self-sabotage like this, or we never get anywhere in life. There are practical things you can do to boost your motivation and keep yourself on track with exercising, like working out with a partner, trying out different types of exercise, rewarding yourself with a TV show or podcast you love afterward, or giving yourself small goals so you have a sense of progress.

You can also reward yourself for keeping it up, whether that's booking in at a fancy spa, buying some new exercise gear, going for a night out, or something else. Some people also enjoy something called the "five-minute rule." This rule states that you have to exercise for five minutes, but if you still really want to quit at that point, you can. It makes it easier to get started (because what's five minutes), and most people will decide to stick at it once they've got over the hurdle of starting. This can help motivate you a lot.

It's also important to think about putting in rest days and recovery days. Rest is crucially important for letting your muscles heal and strengthen. If you're sore, listen to your body and either take a day off or do some gentle exercise (walking, yoga, stretching). Also, remember to switch up what you're exercising, giving some muscles a break while others get their turn to work. You don't do your body any favors by driving it into the ground; treat it with respect, and exercising will be a much more pleasant journey for you.

I can't do traditional movement.

Not everyone is ready to start jogging or hitting the gym. Remember two things: first, it's okay; you'll get there, and second, you can still move. Choose low-impact, easy exercises, such as biking, yoga, Pilates, or swimming. These will not leave you sore like high-impact exercise tends to and can be much less stressful on your body.

I don't know where to start.

There is a ton of good material, plus amazing communities online. You can access all kinds of workouts (from beginners to pros) for free, and if you find a good, supportive community, this helps enormously. You can find guidance and fitness instructors that will help you with basically any aspect of fitness you need. Don't feel like you're alone!

Also, remember that all of us, even the most skilled, trained, and dedicated fitness buffs, started from square one. We began in the same place, not knowing how to use the equipment, unsure about our bodies, struggling to feel at ease with the process of moving. We know the struggle. Most people in this world are enormously kind and helpful and will be glad to guide you as you start your journey. Don't worry about being a newbie: everyone was new once!

It also doesn't really matter where you start, as long as you're being safe. If you're unsure, talk to your doctor before you begin, and go for gentle exercises initially. Remember, respecting your body is critical. This isn't about punishment or aggression; those things don't sustain a healthy fitness journey. This is about helping your body realize its potential in ways that are kind, effective, and fulfilling. We promise that you can do it and that you will feel amazing when you do.

So, although there is much more that we would love to say about movement and how it has changed our lives, we hope it has given you some starting blocks from which you can launch your own exercise journey. In the next chapter, we will start looking at another tool for recovery: spirituality.

CHAPTER 5

Spirituality

Before starting this chapter, we want to express to readers that when we say spirituality, we're looking at another tool designed to smooth out the sharp edges of life and make your food journey easier—a tool that will make the desperate moments feel a little less desperate. Spirituality looks different for everyone, but it is another resource you can turn to to make it easier to keep living when you feel like all hope is gone.

Spirituality is about connecting with yourself and harnessing the power within you to catapult yourself forward into recovery. A lot of people are hesitant when it comes to talking about spirituality, and if you don't want to engage with this chapter at the moment, you don't have to, but for many people, spirituality is a comforter, a place to turn when life kicks you in the teeth, and nothing else can stem the pain. It gives you a power beyond your own, from whatever source you believe in. There is a kind of comfort that we think can only be found through the spiritual channel, whatever spirituality looks like to you.

In this long journey we're on, we need all the help we can get, which is why spirituality is a key tool in the toolkit, helping us just as the other branches help us. It's one of your anchors, keeping you on the lifeboat, helping you stay out of the water, and giving you the strength to keep charting a course to where you want to be.

Before we proceed, we want to emphasize that spirituality doesn't require religion. Spirituality can be found in a myriad of places, experiences, people, and sensations. What matters is that you find something greater than and beyond yourself and feel a sense of connection with that greatness.

So, what does spirituality do for us? We have found that it does a great many things. Initially, it creates a sense of overall well-being, a "bigger picture" purpose, and a bit of scale and perspective. From that foundation, the benefits flow in a multitude of ways. Better sleep, better self-care habits, lower blood pressure, reduced mortality rates, increased compassion (both for others and for ourselves), better relationships, better self-esteem, and better eating choices. When you feel happy, confident, and safe, you will automatically make better choices because they are based on rationality, not fear.

For many people on this challenging journey of learning to eat better, spirituality helps to bring together all the different threads and provides them with a foundation. It gives you peace, clarity, and structure to your day. Imagine, for example, that you choose to recognize your spirituality by sitting and contemplating your garden for ten minutes before you go to bed. Now, you're clearing your mind, you're sleeping better, and you're more rested, so less likely to crave.

Alternatively, imagine that your spirituality takes the form of mindfulness, and you choose to focus more on the experience of eating, so when you go for your lunch break, you get rid of all distractions and just pay attention to your food. Your connection with your food is enhanced, and you find it easier to make healthy, nutritious choices because you are consciously eating.

Perhaps your spirituality is something you find during your movement, instead. Remember, movement can produce a meditative-like state once it becomes part of your life, and it is a time when some people feel connected with a higher being (of whatever nature). Maybe you walk and pray, or you do some yoga and deep breathing and meditate at the same time.

Regardless of your approach, spirituality is like the thread pulling all of the others together. It's the multitool in your box, the one that underpins the other aspects and gives them strength and surety. At the same time, finding a spiritual place that feels right to you is a deeply personal and sometimes challenging journey. Many people have rejected, lost, and found this sense of connection over the centuries. If you don't feel spiritual at the moment, or if you find it's not serving you right now, that's okay too, just like it's okay to recognize that your sleep habits aren't serving you.

We're going to explore our own journeys with spirituality so you can see how this concept has affected both of us in our recovery, and then we'll look at what you can do to start bringing more spiritual connections and peace to your life, whether that's through organized religion or simply a connection with the world around you.

Jamie: Putting Things In God's Hands

Spirituality and I have had a difficult relationship at times, in part because I used to conflate spirituality with religion, and religion with many negative experiences.

For a long time, I used to believe that I had to push, push, push and showcase, showcase, showcase because nobody else was going to do it for me. As I get older, though, my spiritual beliefs tell me that I'm not the creator of the universe; I'm not God, and I'm not supposed to be running the show. I tried running the show for almost 40 years and made a huge mess of my life.

There were many times when I felt I had been successful. When I felt I *was* running things... but everything was a total mess. There were moments in my recovery journey where I looked smaller, I was winning at my career, I "had it all," and yet my life was a lot harder than it needed to be. My approach to spirituality and to my own identity resulted in a lot of conflict and a lot of transient, broken relationships. There was so much wreckage that came from my own doing, my own efforts to do more than I was meant to do. Even controlling (or attempting to control) others because I thought I was playing God, and I thought I had to. I had taken the reins in my hands; I felt I had to steer. It cost me a great deal.

For me, spirituality and religion are closely tied. Once, I thought they were one and the same; I now know they aren't. I thought you couldn't have one without having the other, and I thought that religion was the only way to express spirituality.

I grew up as a Roman Catholic. Church was a very judgmental place for me as a child, filled with "do as I say, not as I do." Growing up in the '80s and '90s, church scandals were ramping up, and I saw many of those I was supposed to look to for guidance and leadership being brought low. Men who had been given roles of power, men who were meant to guide and protect us, corrupting their positions in every way, taking advantage of the people they were in charge of, disillusioning me with the whole world.

It really turned me off religion. I believed that God was in charge of these very corrupt people and that He only rewarded people who were corrupt with leadership. If His spokespeople were corrupt, God must not be who they said He was.

Combine that with a highly tumultuous childhood, where I experienced a lot of loss - of people, of places, of income, of my sense of self. I felt like I was always waiting for the other shoe to drop, always having the rug pulled from under my feet. It didn't seem like there was any spiritual presence. God was a concept, not a reality, and the concept didn't pan out in practice for me because I couldn't see it anywhere in my life.

Unfortunately, my mom and other family members were very religious, and they followed a God who was punishing and judgmental. Anything you did or chose was subject to judgment and ridicule. If I made any kind of bad choice, something that didn't align with my family's expectations, I would hear that God was going to punish me. Didn't study for a test, didn't pick up my room, didn't do my homework... all of these were worthy of punishment.

I quickly came to associate physical harm with having done something wrong. If I stubbed my toe or bumped my head, it was because I had done something to displease God. Everything was black or white, good or evil, and I ended up submerged in a world of fear where I couldn't bear to do wrong.

By the time I reached my late 20s, I was very much "of the world." I had a growing career, a good income; I had married well, owned a big house, had a big wedding ring - all the things that you think make your life worth living. I "had it all." And yet, there was so much that I was lacking. I lacked a sense of inner peace, a sense of guidance, a sense that there was somebody out there I could rely on. I didn't believe in God - I was vehemently opposed to organized religion at this point - so I sought that peace in other humans, particularly men. I had dated a lot, rushed into marriage, and leaned very heavily on my husband. Unfortunately, my codependent tendencies only attracted codependence in turn.

I didn't understand that God was in charge and wanted nothing but good for me. When I lost my mom at 28 years old, I felt very simply that God was dead to me. He couldn't care for me. He had taken away the only person who would fight for me and always be there for me. There was no coming back from there, I thought. "That's it, I'm done." God was not with me, I thought, and never could be again.

At that time, I was dating my now ex-husband, who is also a former Catholic. We had bonded over our loss of religion and considered ourselves both "of the world." God was not at the center of our marriage—He wasn't even in the same state as our marriage. We focused on materialism, we focused on each other, and we focused our energies on finding meaning in anything that wasn't God.

My body and my health became my God. I started to realize that they were everything to me, and I put the pursuit of physical life first. Gaining a smaller body became my one goal, and I thought it would bring me great happiness if only I could achieve it.

And finally, I did. I reached my desired weight, filled my life with health, and even became an advocate for healthy eating. I had everything I had been pursuing. I'd done it. And I remember standing on a stage with a talk show host, talking to a full audience of people about my success... and still feeling empty. There was a God-sized hole inside me. I stopped and thought, "Okay, what did I do wrong? Because I shouldn't still be feeling so empty."

I looked around me to find out what was missing. I had met my material needs. I had lost weight. I had a wonderful partner who supported me and encouraged me, but none of it was enough. That's when I began stepping outside of that union emotionally, looking for people who would validate me but searching for the validation that only God can give. It was very humbling to constantly be grasping at empty straws.

Once I started that process, I was off the rails when it came to any kind of spiritual practice. I was not myself. I didn't recognize the person I'd become, a person who was seeking emotional and romantic validation from people who were not my spouse. It didn't turn physical, but it didn't have to. I was getting myself into a place where the validation and the love of other people drove me, and I thought it was what filled me instead of food.

It created a new identity: "If I look a certain way, I get this kind of attention, and the attention fills me." I focused all my energy on looking and acting in certain ways, maintaining the image that I projected. I did nothing for my spirit or soul; everything was for my physical and worldly body and my physical and worldly pursuits.

By the time I hit 40, I realized I was in a mid-life crisis, and God was absent. Perhaps I should call it a godless crisis instead of mid-life. My soul was screaming by that point for food, for nourishment. Except all the things I was trying to do to nourish it just weren't working.

My husband and I began to talk about separating. I was totally lost. I didn't want to separate, but I didn't have any other option. I had done so much damage to the marriage; we were so disconnected, and he was past the point of no return. We agreed to amicably separate. "There's nothing here, so I'd better leave," I felt. I didn't want to, though. I wanted to stay, to fix it, to work on it. I didn't feel that leaving my marriage was who I was. At the same time, the louder, more worldly part of me kept saying, "You've got nothing left; you've destroyed this, and you need to go because you don't have any other options."

So it was like I was punishing myself, banishing myself from the world that I had created to find a new world for myself. I began to give away everything I owned. We had a big home filled with stuff in North Chicago, all the things you'd think you'd have in a home, life, marriage. It was a beautiful place to look at, but there was no love inside it... I felt it was a true reflection of me. I had obtained physical attractiveness, but I was empty and hollow as a shell. I had no depth. Similarly, my home had no depth. The objects had no meaning to me. To my husband, they only had financial meaning.

When I started giving the stuff away, he thought I was crazy, but I knew the stuff wasn't bringing us any happiness. I donated, gifted, and redistributed the loveless items, and we downsized, moving from Chicago down to Charlotte, NC. We ended up living in separate rooms, totally disconnected from each other, even though everyone around us thought we were married and in love. Indeed, my whole world at that time became one of disconnection - from my body, from my husband, and from God. NC became a symbol of disconnection for me.

It was at this time that I realized I had no other option, and I needed to connect with God. Although I still didn't figure out in what ways. I thought I was just lacking presence, perhaps meditation, spiritual leadership. I started looking around, reading, listening to theorists, and applying tools, but I kept well away from anything religious. I was fixed upon spirituality and felt it was inherently, irrevocably divorced from religion.

Then Wayne Dyer started quoting the Bible, and at first, I didn't want to listen. When Ekhart Toli began talking about the Bible too, discussing the representation of scripture in real life, and exploring how it applies to awakening and healing. I was shocked and disillusioned. I thought they were spiritual, not religious, and I wanted no association with religion. I didn't want to listen when people said that God has nothing to do with organized religion.

I left my marriage in June 2016 and started a consulting job in Houston. I was utterly lost at the time. I thought I was making the right choice. I thought that separating amicably and seizing a new life with a good body and a great career was the right way to handle it. Everything I did was shallow and meaningless. A small part of me kept screaming, asking, "What are you doing?" but I plunged ahead regardless. By this time, I had sold or given away everything I owned except what fit in my car and 12-13 boxes of kitchen stuff, plates, pans, etc. I went from a 2800 sq ft house filled with stuff down to a handful of things. I thought shedding material possessions would help, and to an extent, I know that I was trying to shed my old self and everything I had stood for.

As soon as I started my new life, I realized I'd made a massive mistake, and I needed to go home, but my ex-husband didn't want that. He wouldn't let me come home.

Home was a big deal to me, and I had lost it. I had lost it after my mom. I had given it away when we left Chicago. I had lost it again when I moved from NC. Looking back now, I see that God was stripping me of all these things so that I could finally see Him. I was blind to Him when I kept my husband in the God seat, when I piled his place up with material possessions. I know that if God had meant for me to return to that home, He would have given my ex-husband the desire to talk and reconcile. He didn't want me to go back, so He didn't put those feelings in my ex's heart.

I spent years stomping my foot and shaking my fists, wondering why it happened, like a child unable to accept that their parent has taken something dangerous from them. It took more than five years for the penny to drop and for me to realize that it wasn't God's will that I should be there. If He had willed it, I would've gone back, we'd have rekindled, reconnected, etc. Much of those five years, I spent trying to find a way back, but there were no roads in, no open doors, no jobs in the area, and no willingness on my husband's part. Our union had become ungodly, and because He loved me, He wouldn't let me return to it.

In Houston, I spent my time grasping at straws, focusing on my body shape, dating here and there, throwing myself into my consulting job, and trying to find meaning in something. I got majorly screwed over by my workplace and found myself in a very dark situation eventually, where my consulting firm cut all their hires loose. Now I was alone in Houston, a place that I had only moved to for the job, with no network, no friends, no support... nothing. It was a huge bottom for me. I was still in excellent shape physically, but mentally, everything was a mess.

I wasn't really in a state to be dating, and for the most part, it was very unsuccessful. I did meet one man who I really liked, who was further along in the divorce process than I was, but I still wasn't ready for anything serious. I felt like I had been totally abandoned in the world.

I found a job in New Jersey and moved again, and the guy checked in with me frequently, asking if I was okay, saying he was thinking of me. We stayed friends, and I had another go at sorting my life out. I had no money and didn't want to ask my ex or take on debt, so even getting to NJ was hard. I sold much of my remaining stuff, loaded up the car, and drove to stay with family until I could scrape together enough money to put down a deposit on an apartment. It was good to spend some time with family and I was very grateful for it, but what I really needed was time alone to heal and to reconnect with God. Unfortunately, even now, I didn't realize that.

I threw myself back into dating. I was convinced another person could solve my issues. I was so lonely; of course what I needed was a relationship. New Jersey gave me many good things; my job was wonderful and I met some lovely people, but I was coming from a place of malnourishment spiritually, and my attempts to date were disastrous. Because of the space I was in, I was connecting with similarly broken people, many of them deceptive and dysfunctional. I even ended up in an abusive relationship that quickly turned into stalking when I tried to step out of it, and I had to get a restraining order. I tried as hard as I could to figure out my life, but I still couldn't see what I was missing.

I stayed in touch with my Houston friend, who was now dating someone else. I remember wishing I could find someone like him in NJ. After a few years there, I had begun to create some stability in my life, and started to rediscover my connection with God. It was a wonderful time. I had missed being a daughter, missed my mom so intensely through the darkest moments, and now, I had something akin to that relationship again. I had stopped dating entirely and found myself in a place where I could connect with God and see His movements in my life, His protection and care, the gifts He had given me, the ways He had redirected me. I had begun to nourish my soul at last, finding solace in a connection that went far deeper than any other I had ever known.

I moved to the beach around this time and fell deeply in love with beach life. Financially, I was more secure, and I felt comfortable with my body, comfortable with my family members, comfortable with my boundaries. I started doing lectures at local hospitals about what long-term recovery from obesity looks like, and I felt much of my life had clicked into place.

The man from Houston called to catch up with me. He was single now and said he thought about me a lot. Was I dating?

I wasn't. I wasn't interested in dating anyone local, but I did want to reconnect with him. He was also very spiritual. His faith was strong, and he walked with God. We connected over that shared interest. At the time, I was very active in my church, and he was there (remotely) for my baptism. I found a lot of peace at that time. I felt so much better, now five years on from my divorce. I felt like things were where they were supposed to be, and I was becoming the person I wanted to be. Christianity made sense to me. I loved how I felt when I lived by its values.

Eventually, I got engaged to my Houston chap and agreed to move back there. I didn't want to go back to Houston, but I did want to be with him. I had never had a relationship like this one before. Why would I wait? Unfortunately, I hadn't finished learning my lessons yet.

When I moved back to Texas, I left behind my life of spiritual presence and spiritual growth. I adored my new husband, but I soon found that once more, God's seat was filled by the wrong being—once more, I had placed a man there. It was the wrong thing to do. Wonderful though he was, he was human, not God. He could never meet my needs the way that God could. The codependency I felt was unhealthy.

We went from a place of deep connection and understanding to a place of bickering and anger and many threats on my part about leaving. I was following patterns that I knew, re-making mistakes I had already made. The unhealed parts of me showed up, and his unhealed parts showed up too. We triggered each other constantly, brushing up against the holes and bruises. We stopped putting God at the center of the marriage and put our own needs first.

It was a huge test of faith, and it took so much effort for me to figure out how to stay in the marriage and start facing those wounds. I turned to counseling and began to work on more intensive recovery, trying to heal some of the damage that went right back to my childhood. It was immensely helpful. I learned a lot, uncovered pains I hardly knew existed, and started figuring out how to fix them. I allowed myself to feel much of what I had put away in the past. I learned not to condemn myself or others but to find forgiveness and to try to do something different.

I put down the baggage of the past and started trying to behave in the ways that I knew God would want me to behave. Punishment, self-judgment, self-hatred; all the things I had been trying to shed for so long but had been unknowingly packing up and carrying with me every time I moved... I put them down. I realized that the way to resolve these things, to get rid of the regrets, is to make living amends and to learn. I made sure that my life began to look the way God would want it to. It was the only way I could make up for my past. Guilt, shame, anger, and resentment weren't doing it. They were just making the bags heavier. Behavioral changes let me put the bags down.

I had to be very realistic about how I approached my past. I had to use conviction instead of condemnation and focus on what I could do now rather than what I could have done before. Life got better, and I found the healing process a wonderful experience. Together, we worked on our marriage, worked on healing, and managed to put God back in His place as our guide and our pivot. Our world, which had been askew, pulled back into shape again. It was like getting the oxygen back.

Finally, RFR entered my life. I moved for a work opportunity that would carry me back to New Jersey, which I had really wanted for a long time. Other challenges were waiting for me, though, as they always are. I ended up wooed by the new job, by the world, by my ego, and by the success that I had been waiting for. Within just 3 months, I ended up focused on everything but God. I was so sure of myself, so proud of all I had achieved, so focused on me. Other things, God's place... you know the story. It never ends well.

I have spent the last year unraveling that and re-walking the lessons I learned before about keeping God in His rightful place in my life. In terms of the spiritual part of my recovery, I feel that I've been late to the game, but nonetheless, I'm at the table now. I have gotten here, and perhaps with more experience and more solid lessons than I would otherwise have had. I now know to watch my ego, to watch my attraction to the material, physical world, to the people and places that I want to idolize because I know that when I let this happen, I lose.

It has taken me a long time to figure out where spirituality and religion belong in my life. Determining what God wants vs. what I want vs. what the world wants has been an ongoing challenge. It has pushed me into the water more times than I care to count. When I listen too much to what I want and what the world wants, I end up in a bad place full of heartaches and headaches, disappointments, frustrations, and grief. When I listen to what God wants I heal, I find nourishment, and I find peace.

I know that my recovery is incomplete without spirituality. I had reached physical recovery, a healthy weight, good sleep routines, optimum exercise, and all the rest long before I managed to turn my hand to this tool. Despite being on the lifeboat physically, my mind was still in the ocean. I was still submerged in doubt, struggling against the waves, often trapped in a storm. I needed this key to find a place of calm.

Now, I know that if I spend time with God and prioritize my spiritual practices, life is a lot easier and gentler. It flows. I can stay on the recovery path without having to grip it with my fingernails. I don't have to think about every little move; I don't have to chart the course. I can put my focus on controlling the little things - like food - and trust that God has the rudder and is steering with care. I am not in charge, and it's ludicrous to think that I am. God is.

It took me a lot of lessons to get to this understanding. Ten years of my life, at least, have been spent on it. I kept piling new things into the wrong places, and God kept stripping them away so that I could focus on what mattered: Him. The biggest lesson of all to me? He keeps doing it.

There is great comfort in knowing that you have a captain on this journey and that you are being kept safe. I craved that comfort very deeply over the years, with no knowledge of what I was missing. Now that I have it, I plan to keep it. Without spirituality, your lifeboat will be caught in perpetual storms, and while you might manage to stay aboard, it will be so much harder than it has to be. When you turn to spirituality, you invite calm into your life, and you can breathe more easily.

Paige: God On The Inca Trails

Spirituality was always in my life, from my very earliest memories. I have always felt a connection to God and found solace in this.

Does that mean life was easy for me?

Hell, no. But I had a place to turn when the ugly was unbearable, and I have kept that place throughout the years, taking refuge in it when I am heartsore and exhausted. That said, there have been moments when my spirituality has been tested at the deepest level, where I have found myself punched in the face and reeling from the blow. Those moments have really defined my relationship with Heaven, and those are the journeys I want to share with you.

The first was when Terry, my dad's wife, died. I remember him tapping me on the shoulder sometime around 6 a.m. I knew, even as I surfaced into the conscious world, what he had come to tell me. I got up from the couch and plodded upstairs to where they had turned a sitting room into a makeshift hospice, with the hospital bed right in front of the large picture window. Mother Nature had created a beautiful backdrop of artwork, the garden bursting with fall colors during those final weeks.

My dad's wife had been battling a very rare form of ocular cancer for the past 10 years. She had lived longer than anyone in documented history, even making it into the pages of medical books. She was only 57 (just two years older than me at the time) and had suffered far more than any person should have at that age.

As I pulled up a chair next to the bed to say my final goodbyes, I paused to consider the deeper things in life. It was still dark outside on that cool Kansas morning in late October. I could hear my dad, somewhere else in the house, making the obligatory phone calls.

What came into my heart at that moment was just to sit with her and soak in the first break of sunlight, starting to peek through the dusk. It was important to me that she not be alone in that moment - strange what passes through our minds after someone dies. I couldn't help but wonder what was happening on the other side, and I hoped she wasn't scared. Everything I had learned led me to believe it was a beautiful experience, though.

The silence in the room lent itself to thinking about the essence of these major life moments, followed by the curiosity about how loved ones are able to stand upright in the face of such trauma. As I pondered, it became clear that having a spiritual base allows for grief and comfort to simultaneously coexist in the heart at the exact same point in time. We have all heard the saying that life happens for you, not to you, but when tragedy strikes, that sentiment seems a little hard to swallow. What about the death of a loved one is "for you"?

Whether the sentiment is true or not, who am I to say? But here are the truths that I do know. I know life comes with pointed edges, and when I am active in my spiritual place, it has the power to smooth them out. Spirituality does not mean that we are immune from suffering; it just allows us to experience pain with rose-colored glasses on. I have learned that if I am not prepared in advance and have no place to turn when the chips are down, the ugly starts to come out.

My number one goal is to have a calm brain, and my spirituality plays a big role in maintaining that equilibrium. A spiritual practice offers me a framework for navigating the next step. It provides solace, instills hope and resilience, and allows for perseverance and perspective through hardships. But the biggest benefit of my daily spiritual connection is the opportunity to feel connected to a higher power that can offer a sense of peace and assurance that I am not alone in my struggles. Humans need to feel seen, heard, and understood, and if we rely on others to make us feel significant, we often end up disappointed. Turning to a higher power gives you a sense of reliable, steady, constant comfort, even if it's from a source that is only experienced by the soul.

This is what God looks like to me. Spirituality is the art of letting your mind rest, allowing you to commune with God.

So, when has having faith in my pocket, as a tool at my disposal, been of the most value to me? It was when I was traveling in 2015. Sixteen women were heading out to hike over 50 kilometers and see one of the seven wonders of the world: Machu Picchu.

It was more remote than I could ever have imagined. I was a speck of sand in a world that was suddenly vast. If something had happened out there, in the middle of nowhere, I would never have been found. I remember looking at the llamas grazing on the mountain pastures, the villages where nothing has changed for hundreds of years. It was steeped in kindness but so different.

The physical challenge of climbing Machu Picchu was one of the greatest I have ever undertaken - including my Grand Canyon expeditions. The scenery was among the most beautiful I have ever experienced, and as we walked the Inca Trail, I felt very close to God.

We hiked 40 kilometers in four days, heading up and down mountains, visiting Inca sites, and finally finished on the fourth day at the Sun Gate. From there, we headed down to Augas Calientas to spend the night. A 30-minute bus ride the next day took us to the actual site of Machu Picchu, and from there, some of us decided that we would climb Huayna Picchu - a 9,000-foot mountain. It was the most difficult climb I have ever done, and every step left me exhilarated and full of a sense of purpose.

We then took the last bus ride back down to Aguas Calientes… and the true journey began. The bus driver took us only part way and insisted we get out. None of us spoke his language, so we got off the bus, very confused, and made our way to the village on foot. At that point, things became clear. We were right in the middle of a political protest, with an angry mob of people shouting, screaming, and beating drums in the streets. From what I understand, the government wanted to sell off the rights to some of the Inca Ruins to other countries, and the people were protesting against it.

Immediately, unease set in. I have blonde hair, blue eyes, and was in American attire. I didn't speak the language. I definitely stood out. I now realized why the driver wouldn't come into the city. I didn't know if I was actually in danger, but fear spread quickly through our group. It seemed things could easily get out of control.

Unsure what to do, we walked the streets, trying to find somewhere to get some food after our long morning of hiking. The restaurants were closed out of fear of the protestors. None would be seen feeding Americans. We were potential targets.

After about an hour, a restaurant owner poked his head out and waved me and three others inside with a frantic "Hurry, hurry, hurry." We were ushered into a darkened back room, where we were told to get down and be quiet because there were protesters marching down the alley right in front of his establishment. We had no idea what would happen to any of us if we were caught. My heart was pounding.

Fortunately, the mob passed and didn't return. We were fed quietly and then let out the back door. I pray for that man, and I hope no harm befell him for what he did.

We made a beeline for our hotel, intent on getting the heck out of town, but there was no way out of town except by train, and the train had gone on strike because of the protest. We now had no option but to hike 15 kilometers along the deserted train tracks in the middle of the Peruvian jungle, along the Urubamba River, to a spot called the Hydroelectric plant. Here, we were told, two vans would be waiting and would drive us for seven hours through unpaved mountains back to Cusco.

We set off. At three points during our walk, the tracks passed over rushing streams, and we had nothing to stand on but two narrow planks around a foot apart from each other. I could do nothing but pray I wouldn't fall. At one point, the woman in front of me almost lost her balance. In seeming slow motion, I watched her windmilling her arms wildly. I held my breath since I was right behind her and had nowhere to go but down. If we had fallen, that would have been the end. There was no help nearby. We were on our own.

To make things worse, we were on a deadline. We had to get to the vans before the sun went down, or we'd have been left in pitch blackness. Running out of time, we had no option but to take a shortcut in the last half hour - which meant fighting our way through the jungle on a steep dirt path. I fell twice and once ended up grasping at reeds and underbrush to prevent myself from sliding down a cliff. My knee twisted, and my hip ached.

Finally, we broke free and found the two vans waiting for us. Quickly, we were bundled in. Our guide was not in my van; instead, I was wedged between two men in the front seat and uneasy as I didn't know either of them, nor did I speak their language. We then had seven hours ahead of us, of twisting and turning on dark, remote mountain roads - filled with roadblocks that had to be skirted. The protesters wanted to block every road, and we hit more and more obstacles. We'd see small rock walls, fallen trees, or tire blockades that had been piled up across the path, and we'd have to take another route. Fear welled up in me with each one we met. The local people did not want us here. I was highly concerned they might retaliate because we were using the roads.

We were pulled over by the police at one point. I listened to them talk to the driver and watched them shine a flashlight in the van. I had no idea what they were saying. Our driver was asked for papers, which he produced. I prayed that we would safely pass. Please, let us safely pass. We were in the middle of nowhere, and I knew that if something went wrong, nothing could save me.

We were allowed to move on.

We finally got to Cusco about midnight. There were protests even here, but we were finally back at our hotel. The next morning, Friday, was to be our last day in Peru. I tried to shake off the fear of the night before and enjoy the last few hours. We did some shopping and I used up almost all of my Peruvian money since I wouldn't need it anymore. We enjoyed a nice lunch. I was very ready to head back to the airport, and we went a little early, as we were anxious to get home. In spite of the pleasant day, I had had enough and was ready to leave.

We reached the airport at around 4 p.m., and we were told it was closed. The place was in pandemonium. There had been a crash, and they didn't have the equipment to clear it. I remember the surreal moment when I looked out at the airstrip and saw a guy with a broom and dustpan on the runway, sweeping up the wreckage. It was like watching a guy trimming his lawn with scissors (something I literally witnessed once in Mexico).

No flights were leaving on Friday, and possibly not even on Monday. I had never wanted to get out of a place so badly in all my life. The fear of the night before came back, redoubled, and I was struggling to control my emotions. I had never had a panic attack before, but I thought I might have one then.

Nobody knew what was happening, and no one was in control. Frantic, we contacted our tour guide company, desperate for help. I came up with the idea of renting a bus to drive us to Lima, where our connecting flights were. We wouldn't make it home Friday, but perhaps Saturday. I was already going to be out of my medication, and I had very little money on me.

After several hours of chaos, we were taken back to our hotel, and a bus was arranged. It would take us overnight, across 1,100 kilometers, over mountain passes to Lima. We were told it would be at least 16-18 hours. It actually turned out to be 24 hours. We left at 9:45 p.m., complete with two drivers and a man from the tour guide company, driving at around 20-30 mph. I was in the front seat and I could see absolutely everything: hairpin turn after hairpin turn on unpaved mountain roads, in the darkest of dark. We weren't allowed off the bus until 7:30 the next morning. I drank nothing, and I know God helped me even here. Despite normally using the bathroom a couple of times per night, I made it through.

Those first ten hours of horrible roads were over, but then we hit the desert. Ten more hours of hot, sweaty, unairconditioned driving, with dirt and dust blowing in the windows. Another bathroom break at 12:30.

We got to Lima at 7 p.m. and spent two hours lost in the worst traffic I have ever seen—horns blasting, brakes being slammed on, speeding, lane-crossing—everything mixed together. I have no idea how we didn't get into a wreck, and I was praying the possibility away every moment.

Our driver tried to get a cab to lead us to the airport but failed. Eventually, he found a stranger who agreed to ride with us until we reached the airport. At last, we were there, and gratitude flooded me. I would get home, at last, at last! We were told to get off the bus, grab our suitcases, and run for the terminal. By then it was Saturday evening, and freedom seemed so close I felt I could taste it.

By this time, most of the others had made flight arrangements, or spoken to partners who could do it for them. I'd had no cell service at any point. I knew my husband would be frantic. I had no plan but hoped they could sort it out for me once we were inside. When we got in, though, I realized that everybody except me had a flight out. I was going to be left on my own.

I went to the desk of the airline we were using, and they told me I wasn't in their system. My heart just dropped. After 15 minutes, they found me but told me I would be looking at a $300 flight change charge, and I would have to wait until Monday. Most of my friends had already left, and the rest would be gone soon. I was on my own; I had been awake for over 24 hours, and I had no money left. I couldn't speak the language, and I felt immensely traumatized by what had just happened. I was in a country where I knew I wasn't welcome. I was defeated, dirty, hungry, and emotionally spent like I had never been at any other time in my life.

If you had told me my story before I did it, I would not have believed I would have survived this far. I hated the torment of not knowing what was coming. I was terrified.

I broke down at the LAN counter and began to cry violent sobs. Apparently, hysteria gets action. I was taken behind the counter and walked to a backroom, then handed a phone that connected me with American Airlines in America. As soon as I heard his voice on the other end, I felt safe. He represented everything that was important to me. He was my lifeline. He was a real, live person who understood me; I was one of him. He automatically knew what holidays I celebrated; he knew I watched fireworks on the Fourth of July, and that Americans love the halftime show of the Super Bowl, and cry at the commercials. He was home. I knew he knew our patriotic sentiment that we don't leave people behind. However, he did have to say, "Ma'am, you are going to need to stop crying. I'm trying to help you," but I couldn't stop. I was having a meltdown of epic proportions that was way overdue!

Somebody gave me a cup of water as he began to talk about my options. Eventually, he managed to get me on a plane the next morning, even though all the flights were full.

I will never forget his voice as he told me, there's a flight leaving at 8:10 a.m. "Whatever you do, be at the American counter at 5:10 a.m. when they open. Be the first in line to get your boarding pass. I am booking you, but all the flights are oversold, and if you want out of that country, you must be the first in line."

I can repeat his words perfectly to this day. They ingrained themselves in my mind. He was looking out for me, fighting for my safety, and I was going to heed his advice.

So now I had tickets, but it wasn't over yet. It was 10:30 at night, and I had nowhere to go. I had to stay up for another almost seven hours, before my counter opened, and I was already out of fumes, nothing left to run on. I was in the part of the Lima airport that anybody could come and go from, and I couldn't go into a secure, safe space until I got my boarding passes... at 5 a.m.

Before me loomed one of the darkest nights of my life. I felt like I had given all that I had. Nobody I knew was here. One of my friends had warned me about a pickpocket earlier. I was mentally, physically, and emotionally exhausted, not to mention frightened out of my wits. And under it all, I could feel the fatigue setting in.

I found a Starbucks, bought a large drink and a sandwich, and sat in a corner. I put my backpack behind me and draped my legs over my suitcase, and stayed there for 5 hours. I kept telling myself, just 10 more minutes, just another 10 minutes. Just manage it another 10 minutes. It got me through the night until gastric distress finally took hold at about 4 a.m. At least that gave me something to do!

That night gave me a new, complete understanding of my faith. God doesn't meet you halfway. He meets you all the way, wherever you are, even when you have nothing left to give. I was completely depleted, and I will never know how I made it through that night except that He was with me.

After I staggered out of the bathroom at 4 a.m., I paced and paced until 5 a.m., fighting to stay awake so I could get to the American Airlines counter. My heart was running a marathon in my chest as I waited to hear if a boarding pass was available. It was the last barrier between me and home. If they didn't have it...

But they did. At last, I could go to a safe place inside the terminal. I had to get somewhere with Wi-Fi so I could use my phone to keep myself awake. I still had to keep going until 8:10! Without something, I knew I wouldn't make it.

I had 11 and a half soles left in my pocket and knew I would need to buy something to use the Wi-Fi. I found the only open place was an enormously expensive sushi place. I sat at a table and scoured the menu, only to find everything was 50-60 soles. I asked the waiter if there was anything I could get to eat with what I had left.

He said he could only offer me tea, and I asked if there was anything at all I could eat. He thought about it, and then said, "How about toast?"

I said I would give him everything I had for a piece of toast. I dropped every last coin into his cupped hands. I asked for the Wi-Fi password, and he said there was no Wi-Fi, but I could use one of their computers.

I sank into the seat in front of the computer and watched the screen light up. I was so tired and I had nothing left but this was a safe place I could sit and fight off the fatigue until the plane was ready.

The computer didn't end up working, but the waiter brought me not only one piece of toast but two pieces of toast, plus butter and strawberry jam and a big glass of water. Food had never tasted so good. I gobbled it down with such gratitude, and it seemed to give me the energy boost I needed to make it through the next two hours. I started the 10-minute game again, fighting to keep myself awake. I could hardly believe it when it was actually time to go to the gate.

When it came, I decided I would slip myself through to the first group because all I wanted was to get on the plane. Unfortunately (and not surprisingly, I got called out and had to take the walk of shame past all the A-listers to the C-group). I was aware of my disheveled appearance. I hadn't washed, combed, or deodorized in over 48 hours (and for anyone who knows my level of vanity you will know this was the ultimate level of humiliation - trauma or no trauma).

In spite of all that, when I finally got on the plane, I sank into my seat and quietly wept a prayer of thanks. He had been with me all night, holding my hand. He had been on the phone call to America. He had kept me safe; He had organized food for me. Every one of my other recovery tools and calming mechanisms - good sleep, good food, good exercise - had been stripped away, which only left my spirituality to protect me.

I fell fast asleep while the plane was still on its runway, waking only briefly over the next seven hours. I had a couple of hours of layover in Miami before flying to Dallas. I slept on the plane again on my last flight from Dallas to Wichita.

When I got off the plane and saw my husband, I collapsed in his arms, sobbing with relief, even though I was acutely aware of my appearance and embarrassed by my state. I have never been through such an experience again, and I hope I never have to. When I was finally home and had time to process and reflect, I realized how blessed and protected I had been. I might easily never have made it home. I push away the flashbacks of that time and remind myself that I know I am stronger now because I have discovered what it looks like to walk on the brink.

So, what has religion given me overall? Ultimately, a place to turn when the chips are down, and when you are utterly alone, divided from those around you even by language. I was unreachable by anybody who cared for me, not knowing for sure if I would be on the plane, utterly unrested, and still forced to function if I had any hope of escaping the predicament. I know that as I sat on the airport floor, as I ate the toast, as I waited through those interminable hours, I was being aided by God. I could not have done the task alone. That day, more than any other, defined my relationship with Heaven, and I have never been so grateful that I had already laid the groundwork and created channels of communication so that when I needed help of an otherworldly kind, I knew where to turn.

The RFR Takeaways

What Is Spirituality For You?

The one thing that everyone should recognize about spirituality is that it is unique to each of us. We aren't here to tell you to believe in the Christian God or any other God. All we want to do is teach you that spirituality is part of a cohesive life, whatever form it takes. It nourishes you, it restores you, and it serves as a final shield when life throws rocks your way.

But what shape and form spirituality takes and how you practice it are up to you. We just want you to have it as part of your arsenal, one more tool to keep you on the lifeboat, another anchor in the storms. For many people, spirituality is a source of calm... and remember that calm minds don't crave.

Many people don't know how to incorporate spirituality into their lives, though. Here are a few suggestions that might help.

Join A Community

Not everybody wants to share their spirituality with others, but if you are inclined to do so, you may find great joy in this. Spiritual communities can give us deep connections and support networks, sometimes greater than any other kind of network. You may find opportunities to volunteer or to get help if you need it, and you may form valuable connections with those around you. Any and all of these things can help you find spirituality and make it part of your life.

Meditate

Meditation is often sneered at because it is hard to practice. In today's ever-busy world, taking time to sit and do nothing, letting your mind turn, feels unnatural to many of us. However, meditation has been linked with many health benefits, and it offers you an opportunity to let yourself simply be in the present moment, whatever that moment is.

Meditation doesn't have to be about sitting and staring into space or chanting the way it is often depicted in the media. You can meditate while walking around the block or exercising, or just take a few minutes to breathe deeply and focus on your body before you go to sleep.

Spend Time Reflecting

Time for reflection often helps us to connect with our spiritual selves. Notably, we often feel least like doing this when we need it the most. When things are bad, we try to put them aside and focus on the good, but taking a few minutes each day to think about what went well, what went better, and how we could have changed it can be key to making life choices that are right for you. Reflecting on the good things and feeling how fortunate you are will often help you to feel more connected with a higher power and give you a sense of perspective that can be hard to achieve in the day-to-day rush.

Pray

You don't have to pray in the traditional fashion if this isn't speaking to you, but sometimes, speaking to another being that you trust and talking to them about your problems can be freeing. Prayers can take many forms, whether you write your thoughts, keep them in your head, or speak them aloud, but you know what they say: a problem shared is a problem halved. We don't always want to share our problems with the people in our lives, but we can always share them with a higher being, and there is something immensely comforting in that.

Spend Time In Nature

Many of us forget the power that nature has to make us feel part of something bigger. Standing on a mountain, listening to a waterfall, marveling over a forest - all of these things help us connect with the world around us and find our places in it. The sights that make you feel small and take your breath away are those that are the most powerful, but you don't have to go to Machu Picchu or see the Northern Lights or explore the jungle for these things... you just have to spend a bit of time remembering how breathtaking the natural world is.

Taking the time to watch and enjoy nature is crucial for our mental well-being and our spiritual journeys. There is enormous peace to be found just in watching a trail of ants or admiring a flower. We can all tap into this resource in different ways, and we should make space for it as much as possible. Walk in the park, stand in a garden, or even just grow some indoor herbs and marvel over the process from seed to plant. All of these things will bring you peace and spiritual meaning.

Hopefully, you now have a sense of what spirituality can provide as a tool and an anchor in the food addiction challenge. In the next chapter, we will start looking at stress management and emotional intelligence, helping you suss out how these two aspects play into healthy eating.

CHAPTER 6

Stress Management in an Emotionally Intelligent Way

How do you handle stress? If you're like most people and if we're going to be honest... not great. That's why stress management and emotional awareness are two important branches of our program.

Stress is one of those things that we all live with. It's part of the human experience and not one that we can (or should) try to eliminate entirely from our lives. That said, most of us would agree that the world we live in can be unnecessarily stressful at times and that we are forced to cope with sometimes inordinately high degrees of stress for extended periods. Humans are pretty decent when it comes to coping with short-term stress, but once stress becomes chronic, we run into a whole range of issues.

You may already know that stress isn't good for your health, but you might not realize just how many problems it can cause. High blood pressure, heart disease, and obesity are just a few on the list. And yes, stress really can make you overweight because the high cortisol levels encourage fat storage and increase your insulin levels. That also increases your risk of diabetes. It's easy to see how these issues put you at risk of serious diseases and problems like heart attacks.

What's more, ongoing stress invites difficulty when attempting to make responsible food choices. Many of us turn to food for comfort when we are uncomfortable, and we opt for foods that are high in sugar, salt, and fat because these make us feel - temporarily - better. When we do this, we are giving food a bigger job than it was ever designed to do. As we've seen in previous chapters, we're abusing food when this happens because it's no longer about nourishment.

It's also worth noting that women often shoulder more stress than men because of childcare (or other care) responsibilities and household chores being combined with the stress of work, whereas men more often can just focus on work. That's not a hard and fast rule, of course, but it's worth bearing the generalization in mind as you figure out your own relationship with stress.

Add anxiety and depression to the list of problems that stress causes and it becomes clear why stress management is another of the important branches of our tree. So, let's start exploring our experiences with stress management and go from there.

Jamie: Stress in Mind, Stress in Body

I've spent most of my life steeped in anxiety. Growing up in a tumultuous environment and burning my way through a series of pretty debilitating challenges in my teens and twenties means that life has given me plenty to stretch my anxiety muscles over. I also saw enormous amounts of anxiety (and poor coping mechanisms) modeled for me in my early life, and I assumed that was just the modus operandi for most people.

I realized that stress was a problem for me in college, when the stress of a new environment, driving, managing money, and being away from home meant I found myself uncomfortable in my own skin and in everything I was doing. I had always used food to manage anxiety, and no other coping mechanisms had ever been taught to me. Nobody showed me how to manage emotions or create emotional intelligence. Being told to relax or being shamed for the feeling was far more common. I had no idea how to process my emotions, and I found myself with all kinds of negative behavioral traits; I jumped to conclusions, I got frustrated, I lost my temper.

Leaving college didn't make things better. I was even more exposed to the big wide world, even more anxious about money, living alone, and taking the first steps of adulthood. I joined a community that essentially served as a continuation of college, and that made a big difference; I was taking the same steps as those around me: buying my first car, renting my first apartment, starting my career, and testing the waters with my first real relationship.

We grew into adults together and that helped me enormously. Here, I learned my first stress management tool: community. Support from others who can truly empathize is invaluable. It helped an indescribable amount, and it did a lot for me... until I lost my mother. After that, I was plagued by constant stress and grief and had no community to turn to and no buddy to pair with. Food was the only thing I could find to fill the gap. At that point, I wasn't even using it for stress management. I was using it like a numbing drug that took away the pain and let me breathe again.

That led to an enormously tumultuous period, where I was still going through the motions of young adulthood, but my life was constantly colored by anxiety. Everything in my life except food felt wrong. Or, maybe I was wrong. I was really struggling to cope.

A few years after my mother's death, I realized my life was being run by stress, so I went to counseling and began the proper process of grieving - both for my mom and for other losses. I came to recognize many good things during this period, including finding my connection with God. I began to see that He was protecting me. The counseling helped with my weight loss journey too; I started to feel better, to feel heard and seen and understood. My counselors helped me connect again, and I really appreciated that journey, which then led me to fitness and to the gym community I described earlier. Another community to share these early steps with!

I still suffered from anxiety, but now I had more tools for managing it. Food, I gradually noticed, was no longer one of them. It was a great feeling while it lasted, but then my anxiety began to take shape in a new form. I realized that I didn't know how to be married. I didn't know how to form a successful partnership. I didn't know how to "be" within the life I had created for myself.

I used the tools I'd been taught, but as you'll know from the last chapter, it wasn't enough to save my marriage. I packed up, left, and found myself alone in Houston. Totally alone. And alone is not good for me. There was no "divorced and vulnerable women's community" waiting for me. I ended up feeling sorry for myself, enormously disconnected, and very stressed by what had happened. Many of my tools fell apart, and I turned back to food. I began using it in unhealthy ways again and developed a binge-eating, bulimia approach in an attempt to exert some control over my life.

I did keep trying with my other tools; I joined a gym and began making friends, and I tried to go out and socialize when I could. I had to be careful with money, though. A couple of the things that I found lowered my anxiety was making sure I met my basic needs and focusing on how to get my career back on track.

And then my move to New Jersey came, and as you might guess from the previous chapter, things got better. My personal life stayed rocky, but closer to family and with a new job in hand, I could use my stress management tools in more effective ways. I also developed a lot of new tools, and I could feel my coping mechanisms evolving with my recovery. Even more, I was at a low-stress point, with my comfy little beach town, my connection with God, my spirituality, my church community, family and friends nearby... and then COVID-19 knocked me flat on my back again.

I don't cope well with being alone, in case you haven't noticed from the recurring theme of community throughout my story. Before we all began doing the Zoom thing, it was just me and my dog. Even with Zoom, those first few months were really rough. I felt like the pandemic of COVID would soon be replaced with a pandemic of depression and loneliness. I need connections to feel okay, and so do many other people. When you look at the aftermath of the pandemic years, I don't think my predictions were far off.

When I started dating my now-husband, things improved again. I discovered that having an exciting event on the horizon really helps me handle stress. My move back to Houston and marriage helped a lot. I still had to remake many connections and rebuild large parts of my life, but the precautions in Texas were less stringent; I could go out (masked) and get to know people. I again reached a healthy weight, and my anxiety eased.

Next came another curveball. I was offered a promotion in New Jersey, and we devised a plan for me to split my time, half the year there and half in Houston. I got a New Jersey place and plunged in with enormous excitement, only to find that things just weren't great. I started getting sick. A lot. Over and over again. I put it down to missing my husband, or to not being used to the weather. It got worse as time passed. I was fatigued all the time. I was exhausted and drained. I couldn't keep up, and my stress was constantly escalating.

And then I didn't get the promised promotion. It was handled badly, and at the time, I was very hurt. It actually turned out to be a godsend - and proof that He is always looking out for me, and He will give me things that are meant for me. A month and a half after the promotion failed to come through, there was a storm. The ceiling began to leak. I remember watching the water flood down in a sort of numb horror, and then rushing to get my stuff out. The rest is a blur of motion, anxiety, and pure panic.

For a few days after that disaster, I tried to keep things running in NJ, but nothing was working. In the end, I drove back to Houston because I knew that what I needed more than anything was to be with my husband. I got back five days after the flood and just slept. I slept and slept. At the time, I thought it was exhaustion from the stress, but afterward, I discovered that I was going through perimenopause.

Even that wasn't enough of an explanation for everything. I was getting a lot of stress responses from my body, mostly related to physical stress (I had the emotional stress management down pat by this point!). I became very sensitive to both my environment and my food. I started getting swelling and bad reactions. I couldn't think straight. I had brain fog, fatigue, and irritation. It wasn't just midlife. It wasn't just stress. Something was wrong.

My husband eventually sat me down and said I didn't seem myself and that I was in the wrong headspace. I knew something was wrong, but I didn't know what. No matter how much I slept, how much time off I took, or what I ate, I didn't feel good.

I got in touch with my doctor and they eventually identified major liver function issues, meaning that, basically, I was constantly having an immune response. I had to move onto an elimination diet of just meat, water, and greens. I'm still eating that at the time of writing. I was okay with the change because the alternative was unlivable... but things were still wrong. I gained 30 lbs in just 3 months, and I got very frightened. I knew something else was going on. I tried again, different doctors, different diagnoses... and eventually, I found my way to a nutritionist. She asked me if I had been exposed to mold at some point, and the penny dropped.

It hadn't just been a leaky ceiling on that one night of the storm. It had been leaking for months. I had been breathing in moldy air, my ceiling fan spreading it about my room, filling my home with poison. I had mold toxicity. I'd had a nagging feeling, a faint suspicion, but both I and those I'd raised it with had brushed it aside. It was just a leaky ceiling, after all... except that it wasn't. And the damage was huge.

Now, I've started a protocol to bind and detoxify. I'm having to learn how to manage both my daily mental stress and my physical stress. I'm having to reverse all the tricks I used in the past that aren't working anymore and find alternatives. I've gone from a purely plant-based diet to almost totally animal-based pretty much overnight. The pressure has been enormous.

Even that change wasn't enough. I had to go on a spiritual journey, pausing and stopping all the noise around me so I could listen to what my body needed. I found that not all animal products agreed with me. Eventually, I settled on locally-sourced, organic foods and began paying close attention to how my body feels.

I also ditched everything toxic from my beauty routine. To some extent, I'm at the extreme right now, but what's amazing is that I am very slowly starting to feel better. The body that I have fought so hard to heal in the past has been broken again, and I'm having to once more figure out how to heal it—but with a whole new set of tools and approaches.

I'm leaning heavily on my faith, my spirituality, and my community throughout the process. I've built a team of people across the globe (literally; my nutritionist is in Australia), and they are all helping me get my health back. I hope that sometime soon, I can step up the gear with my fitness and get that back on track, too - once I've healed. It has been a wild journey, but God has continued to give me what I need and helped me manage the stress and emotions throughout. He has taught me how to let go, surrender, listen to my body, and pay attention to what it needs and doesn't need. Taking the time to rest, slow down, and remove obligations from my life has helped enormously, too.

And the effects are already showing. The inflammation, weight, and autoimmune symptoms are disappearing, and I've lost 20 of the 30 lbs. I'm less tired. I can function better. I'm still a long way from healed and I can't quite tick along as I'd like to... but life's a whole lot better now.

So it seems like life has really done its best to test my stress capacity in every way; I've done emotional and grief-related stress, I've done loneliness and self-doubt, and I've done physical stress in the strangest, most scary of ways. I've gone through the wringer when it comes to handling it. I've figured out that finding communities I can depend upon, retaining my faith, and listening to what my body needs when stress hits are the most powerful ways to combat it. I know there's still a roller-coaster ahead of me, but I also know that those tools will carry me through and give me what I need to cope with these challenges, whatever form they take going forward.

It's been a great reminder that I don't have it all figured out, and I can't rest on my laurels. I need to keep looking in the mirror, listening to my body, and responding to its needs. As our bodies grow and change, we have to change how we care for them. We aren't numbers on a scale, pictures in an album, a face or form in a mirror. We are so much more, so much deeper, and we need to champion that, honor it, fight for it. We need to love ourselves and put nurturing first.

Paige: Power of the Pause

Some people find managing stress and processing emotions comes naturally. Not me. Freezing comes naturally, and emotional processing comes painfully slow. As a child, I would just stand like a pillar of salt when something around me was upsetting or traumatic, my feet cementing themselves to the floor. It was an automatic response, almost reflexive. Then, I would wait for the feeling in my legs to come back so I could move. That would allow the emotion to settle down. Then, I would bury it all deep in the recesses of my organs and go about my business. After all, isn't that what most normal, healthy people do?

That system works great until it doesn't. Hello, adulthood. A place where you have to think faster, solve problems, and, for many of us, be in charge of little people who look at us with laser beams darting from their eyes, demanding immediate answers to problems. Cue the chest tightening and racing thoughts, feeling like a gerbil on a hamster wheel needing to pick up the pace.

Learning how to manage stress was forced on me as life unfolded into college, family, jobs, financial responsibilities, and relationships that were not always easy. There were bonuses to these experiences, of course; they allowed me to practice the skills that would carry over into the unplanned, especially as I found my way into recovery from sugar addiction.

Sugar was a major part of my stress management before recovery. Full disclosure: it was the only tool in the toolbox. One of my earliest memories came at the beginning of my career, back in the '80s, when cookies were how I solved problems. I will tell you now: chocolate chip cookies weren't a want; they were a need.

By second semester of nursing school, I had been assigned to the Veterans Affairs hospital for my very first clinical. From the moment I walked in, that familiar pungent smell of cleaning fluid and other substances hit me in the face with forceful vigor. That's when the ride on the struggle bus started its engine and pulled out of the station. The depressed condition of the building commingled with the tragic cases it housed and I began to feel that floaty feeling washing over me. I was having trouble thinking clearly. Every minute was painful, and hours felt like days. I was in full uniform, I had the qualifications, I looked the part - and yet I felt so out of place that I could barely function. Seeing the condition these people were in, the pain and grief that their loyalty had bought them was my undoing, and when I could finally get out of there, I knew the only thing that would put me back together was sugar.

I had a pounding headache, my heart hurt, and I was working hard to pull it together enough to get back to campus at Wichita State University and stand in line for my drug of choice. A chocolate chip cookie would solve all the day's problems and take away the sorrow and stress (and supersize it, would ya... I've had a hard day). With the first bite, the desperation melted as I inhaled euphoria, swallowing relief into my veins. Butter, sugar, flour - an amalgamation of peace that only cost $1.29.

If you have never experienced cravings, they feel like a deep throbbing ache gripping the insides of your chest cavity, internally crippling you into the fetal position, driving you to make choices you would not otherwise have considered. It felt like a bargain to sell my soul for a dollar and some coins. Whatever it took to stop the pain.

As always, it was short-lived and followed by a keen awareness of what I was doing, but I couldn't stop; I didn't know how to stop. Didn't really want to stop. To make matters worse, I was no more prepared to go back and face my next shift than I had been before the cookie. I hadn't fixed anything, only numbed myself briefly. They say change is on the other side of awareness. I didn't have the vocabulary then, but almost four decades later, I now recognize that pivotal moment was the start of my journey.

As the years have passed, I have learned that being able to calm oneself is one of the greatest assets any human can possess. It is right up there with emotional intelligence; it is how we learn to trust ourselves. It's the difference between positive and negative outcomes; it's the difference between winning and losing. It shows up in impulse control, which drives your future. When you can remain calm, you can respond rather than react. And if life has taught me anything, it's that calm is never found at the bottom of a cookie jar.

As I have spent time in recovery, stress management has allowed me to develop a "pause button" between thoughts and actions, a small space that saves people from tragic consequences. The button allows rational self-talk to do its job. We change the automatic "I can't" to "I have never done this but I can try." In the pause, you can give yourself a pep talk that will get you through the challenge ahead. This is how winners think, and it is a skill every human can develop. We talk a lot about the things we can control and the things we can't control. Self-talk and re-framing are all superpowers within our control and the key to managing stress and remaining calm.

I mentioned earlier that I climb Pikes Peak every year for my birthday; I will be completing my 13th climb during the writing of this book, and every time, I remember how that pause button has helped me. One year, my climbing group spread out a bit, and I ended up hiking a few miles alone. I don't mind solitude; it is an intensely meditative, spiritual experience. You learn so much on the path: it is as if the earth is speaking wisdom into every fiber of your being with each footstep. There is something about being buried among silent pine trees that allows you to commune with your deepest self.

Of course, it's not so great if you get so caught up in thoughts that you take a wrong turn… and when I stumbled upon that proverbial fork in the road, I zigged when I should have zagged.

Nothing snaps you back into reality faster than realizing you are lost and alone in the woods. I knew it wasn't safe to hike alone. Sure, there were others behind me, so if I broke my neck, someone might be along soon, but that safety net does nothing if you cannot be seen or heard.

What caught my attention was the ground beneath my feet had turned spongy. The strong, firm path that confirmed my safe direction was suddenly gone. I felt myself sinking ever so slightly into marshy earth.

When I realized what I had done, I reverted to my childlike pattern of freezing in place. I began to swallow down panic as life started unfolding in slow motion. In an attempt to calm myself, I activated all my senses, switching into survival mode. I could almost feel my pupils dilating while my ears were perking up, lifting for sound. I told myself not to panic (remember the self-talk I just mentioned). I hit the pause button and let rationality kick in.

Sure, I had food in my backpack, and all that stood between me and temporarily numbing out was a thin, zippered piece of nylon, but I had developed enough skills by this point that I knew abusing food was going to make life a whole lot worse, not better. No one knew I was lost, and no one was coming to save me.

I had to make a plan. I tried to recall how long ago I might have gone off-track. Could I turn around and go back the way I came?

I scanned my surroundings to start negotiating my next move. I wasn't sure if I had traveled in a straight line or at an angle. If I tried to retrace my steps, there was a chance of getting even deeper off track. I needed help. This was bigger than me and I was very frightened. I felt so alone, but I knew that wasn't entirely true. There were plenty of animals - like bears - sharing those trees with me.

On a previous year, I'd seen a cub scamper across the trail right in front of me. That hadn't bothered me, but what might be coming behind that ball of fur certainly did. That time, I also froze, and then, after assessing I was in the clear and momma wasn't coming, I bolted for the summit of the mountain. Despite the fact that I was on my 11th mile at that point, it felt like there were fireworks of adrenaline in my muscles, and I think that might have been my fastest year ever. Stress management at its finest. Used correctly, it can help break records.

Now, though, I was lost in the thicket and unsure of my next move. I was desperate to stay calm and think straight. I started to pray; I knew that would provide some comfort, and hopefully direction. Out loud, as if God were standing next to me, I started to plead for guidance. God, I am lost, I am scared, I might be in danger and I don't know what to do, please have mercy on me and help me find my way. I need your help right **NOW**.

As soon as I finished speaking, the Divine answered me in the form of a thought. I was immediately able to collect myself. I made a quarter turn to the right. I knew the path had to be in that direction. I listened with all my might for far-off voices. They were faintly audible, but I couldn't detect exactly where they were coming from. I repeatedly told myself to be calm. Don't freeze, don't panic. This is a time to rely on your skills. I could plan an emotional bubble bath and process the events of the day when I was out of this mess. I mustered all the bravery I could manage, and took my first step into the unknown.

It was a terrifying process; this part of the woods was wilder and more overgrown than the area we usually walked, and I could hardly believe I'd come so far without noticing it. I was being forced to climb over boulders and fight old, low-hanging branches. After every bob and weave, I would listen, trying to mentally measure if the distant voices were becoming stronger or softer. That feedback would allow me to edit my direction. Finally, after what seemed an eternity, I could pick out conversations, not just muffled sounds. I was suppressing hysteria as I finally popped out of the woods onto the path. I was never so happy to be back on the Barr Trail in all my life - and apologies to the nice couple from Minnesota that I startled half to death with my sudden appearance.

Is this an example of stress management? I think so. What if I had panicked? What if I couldn't think straight? What if I'd told myself, this is too hard? Or if I'd given up? What if I really had sat down to eat instead of to think? I chose to hit "pause" so I could pull myself together, rely on everything I had learned, and work through the process to a logical solution. I could not have done that if I were altered by sugar: I would have been a victim, not a victor.

When you're faced with an obstacle, you can give up, or you can find a way to deal with the wall in front of you. Are you going to climb it, go around it, or dig a hole and crawl under it? Are you going to knock it down and march over it, or are you going to turn around, go home, and pull the covers up over your head?

The great news is, life experience provides the best opportunity to improve your confidence. When you overcome difficult situations, you begin to consider yourself a seasoned pro at handling life on life's terms. Indeed, you're training your brain, creating new neural pathways that confirm you know how to handle this, and you can succeed. Sure, it's not easy, fun, or fast, and there will be setbacks - but it can be done.

It was this kind of training that let me face up to one of the biggest sources of stress I ever encountered: the challenge of giving up sugar, aware that I had failed every other time. Just the thought of trying was overwhelming, but knowing I'd faced other stressors and triumphed made it easier. I could do it - and with my stress management tools, I did.

I kind of want to rename "stress management" to "strategist expert" because that's how I view handling stress: working out how to deal with the situation. You want your default to change from "I can't" to "let me figure this out." Part of that lies in proving to yourself that you are capable and building confidence in yourself so that even when the chips are down (pun intended), you know you've got this and you're in control.

It's also worth remembering that stress can be dishonest, so don't believe what your mind tells you straight away. Reframe the situation, consider it from different angles, and then begin planning your approach. By this time, rational thought will have taken over, and the stress will have begun to dissipate. You can then put your plan into execution! This is the perfect formula to reduce the emotion to an appropriate level.

What's more, it will also help you spot the lies that your brain tells you, like saying that ultra-processed foods will make things better. Was the cookie actually going to make my rotation at the Veterans Affairs hospital less traumatic and stressful? Somehow, take away the grief? Not likely! It's a short-lived solution that perpetuates a vicious cycle, and as my skills have evolved over the years, I've seen through this stress response and found other, genuinely effective solutions.

The RFR Takeaways

How To Build Stress Management and Emotional Intelligence

Of course, you'll find entire books dedicated to these two things, and we obviously haven't got the scope to do that here. Our desire is mostly to draw your attention to how critical stress management and emotional intelligence are when it comes to managing your food addiction. However, we will run through some basics that should help you start.

Think About Control

Stress very frequently centers on what we can and can't control. When we feel in control of a situation, it's not usually a source of stress. A top stress-busting technique involves figuring out what you can and can't control. Once you've come to grips with that, focus on the parts you can control and start building an action plan from there.

Label Your Stress

Don't be afraid to acknowledge it when you feel stressed. We all feel stressed sometimes. We live in a high-pressure world where there's often a lot at stake, and we get worked up. It's okay. Acknowledging that and reminding yourself to take a deep breath and start implementing your anti-stress techniques is a great way to mitigate the stress and start functioning again.

Find Relaxation Techniques

There are hundreds of techniques out there, and it's worth trying a few until you figure out what works for you. Breathing exercises, mindfulness, regular meditation - any of these things can help. Some will help more in certain situations than others. Meditation before bed, for example, might give you a better sense of overall calm, while breathing exercises might help in a tense moment.

Walking, working out, spending time with pets, initiating physical contact, engaging with hobbies, and getting out into nature can all help, too. Remember that you want to mitigate long-term stress as well as short-term bursts, so make sure you put "relaxation" in your regular calendar so you deliberately spend time unwinding and lowering your overall stress.

Make Life Easier

If you're in a period with a lot of stress, remember that it's okay to make life easier for yourself; you don't have to perform at 100% all the time. That might mean letting the house get a little messier, not doing certain chores, or declining favors/extra work tasks if feasible. Whatever cutting yourself some slack looks like, remember to do it when you're stressed!

Sometimes, when we get stressed, we try to force ourselves to perform at our best, as though we have something to prove. Instead, try to let the little things go and make life easier. You can always prioritize what absolutely needs to be done right now and let the rest go until next week when things have calmed down!

In particular, try to make healthy eating easy; you're much more likely to go off the rails if you're trying to cook gourmet healthy meals on top of everything else, so look for simple ways to enjoy good food. An enormous number of vegetables can be eaten raw or simply steamed or baked. Eating well will give you the fuel to cope with stress, so make sure your food doesn't fall off the radar when you're in red alert mode.

Make A Gratitude List

Gratitude lists help us focus on the good things in life, so they're a very effective way to combat stress. Write out the things you are glad you have, even if they feel trivial or unimportant in the bigger picture. When you do this, you teach your brain to look for the positives, which is a great trick for rewiring your thoughts.

Practice The Art Of "No"

Even though most of this chapter has been about recognizing your power and remembering to say "I can" when something challenges you, it's important to realize that it doesn't mean you have to say "yes" to every request that comes your way. Don't want to go to that party, play tennis, work out, go to the cinema, take a stretch project at work, or volunteer at an event? Don't!

Remember, fighting stress is about being in control. We're in control when we say "no" when we don't want to do something, not because it scares us but because we can't complete the task at that moment. Your life will be less stressful if you remind yourself that you have the right to say "No," and you exert that right occasionally.

Help Someone Out

Sometimes, we feel utterly powerless in our lives, but fascinatingly, we can often combat that by exerting our power in other ways. Doing something for another person is an amazingly effective way to overcome our sense of powerlessness and give ourselves a boost. It also helps us remove our focus from our own problems and lets us pay attention to others—one of the surest ways to kick stress to the curb.

Look For Triggers

Understanding your stress response better is often helpful, too. For many of us, stress is an underlying sense that something isn't right. It's not always about the situation that's in front of us, even if that feels stressful because of its immediacy. Following a feeling of stress back to its source can help us handle it more effectively because we can look for the control factors and begin creating a plan of action.

Try to pinpoint trends, too; recognizing the things that often cause stress can help you develop better tools for dealing with those triggers. Do you often freak out at work? If so, is there something you can do to make your career less stressful? Are you worried about your relationship? If so, might counseling help? Trends give us insights that help us tackle stress from a more preemptive and often more powerful position.

Similarly, pay attention to how your body responds to stress, as this offers you further insights into what's going on and how you should handle it. If your chest gets tight, try deep breathing. If you feel faint, sit quietly for a bit.

Check In With Yourself

Not meeting our needs is often a source of stress, but it's important to actually figure out what those needs are before you start trying to meet them. When you feel hungry, it's a sign that your body wants something, but not necessarily food! Before heading to the pantry, take a few moments to check in with your other needs and your emotions. Is your body sending a hunger signal because you're stressed, tired, lonely, thirsty, bored or something else? Ask yourself, what am I really needing in this moment?

You can think of this like a mental hug, where you pause for a few moments and just ask your body what's going on with it and listen carefully to the answer. Be patient and really listen, and you'll soon get to the root cause of your stress, whereupon you can start finding solutions.

Make Your Future Self Your "BFF"

When it comes to handling stress, you have to think of your future self. Stress is often related to what might happen, so we try to protect ourselves from harm. The choices you make in response to a stressful situation will determine what your future self experiences. Making good choices that resolve issues sets that future self up for success and enhances their well-being, so think about them and treat them as the valuable people they are. They deserve it!

Plan Where You Can

Another great motto, "plan where you can" means being as prepared as possible for life in general. It's about making the effort to put your keys in the same place so you can grab them in the morning or fill the gas tank before it's empty so you don't have to do it when you're already late for work.

Basically, if you run your life in chaos mode, you're always slightly stressed, and when a curveball comes, you can't handle it. Your slightly-late-for-work becomes really late and a conversation with your manager - or some equivalent.

This has something in common with the tip to make your future self your best friend. Basically, you take stress out of your future self's life, and you'll find that you deal with far fewer problems overall. You might like to think of this as making deposits into the stress bank account for a rainy day; by taking on that problem now, you don't have to deal with it later, and might give yourself more bandwidth to deal with an unexpected crisis. It's a trick that requires some self-discipline, but it really works, and you'll thank yourself for it when a plan comes unraveled but you can still pull through because you've got your backups in place.

So, hopefully, if we ask, "How do you handle stress in an emotionally intelligent way?" you've got more tools at your disposal and a better approach!

CHAPTER 7

Connection To Self

The whole idea of connection to self is what a healthy relationship with ourselves looks like. Unless you've got a healthy relationship with you, controlling cravings and dealing with addiction can be enormously challenging - maybe even impossible. Sadly, though, many of us don't really understand what connection to self even looks like! We don't spend a lot of time getting to know who we are, and this isn't the sort of thing that schools tend to teach you.

Yet, connection to self is fundamental to recovery. You can't heal yourself, protect and nurture yourself or look in the mirror and see a stranger. It's time to change that. Spending time with your inner family, another branch on our tree, is an important exercise.

The journey to self-discovery can be long and involves many hiccups, but it's only by taking these steps that you can succeed in recovery. You don't want to be on a lifeboat with a stranger, do you? You want to be on a lifeboat with somebody you understand, trust, and accept. We're working toward that in this chapter, so let us share our stories with self-discovery and then look at how you can use them.

Jamie: Baggage in the Attic

I've always been dead from the neck down. I spent most of my life totally disconnected from my body. I disassociated; I rejected it in all ways: for how it functioned or didn't, for what it did or should have done. I was locked away in my head, worrying about the future and the past, thinking about pleasing others, and stressing over what might happen if others didn't do what I wanted.

If that sounds manipulative, it was, but not maliciously so. I didn't realize I was doing it for most of my life and it wasn't for personal gain. I was just so filled with fear I thought I needed to control everything because I didn't trust myself to manage if I wasn't in charge.

Whenever I got caught manipulating people, I would feel ashamed. I knew it was wrong, but I didn't understand why I did it. I didn't recognize that it stemmed from a fundamental distrust of myself, the world, and God. I was disconnected from the loving, kind adult self within me - my true self - and somebody else was running the show.

When I began my recovery journey and found my connection to God, things improved. I began to put my trust in myself and Him, and I realized that He had been there throughout my life, constantly working things out for me, even in my lowest times. I began to trust Him, and at that point, my loving adult self started to show her face. As my recovery continued, I also began to trust that self.

Finally, I could navigate life on life's terms. I began enjoying the ride instead of trying to force myself into the driver's seat. The sense of freedom was euphoric, and I could finally feel connected with myself in the present. It was a very long journey, though.

I had spent around 40 years disassociating from my body because I couldn't stand to be present in the pain my body felt, the pain that drove me to eat. Existing was uncomfortable, and eating numbed that. I didn't even know something was wrong. I thought feelings were just words rather than actual sensations in my body. I didn't know that they were trying to tell me something.

Around 2017, I decided to do a 12-step recovery program on relationships. I thought it was about my relationship with others, but it was really about my relationship with God and myself. I began to see there was a whole inner world I'd disassociated from, many parts of my psyche that I had rejected. These parts were me at different ages. I realized that I had a whole world of "me" inside me that wanted to be seen, acknowledged, and healed.

But how? I had some good parenting examples on my mom's side, but much of my childhood was highly dysfunctional and I had no idea how to "re-parent" myself. There was a lot of work to be done, but once I realized that I could trust God and I didn't have to control everything, I could just sit with myself and begin to connect. It took effort. I had to learn how to co-exist with myself and all the stuff I had going on emotionally and physically so that I could get to know myself.

It was like learning all about a stranger... and it opened the door to all kinds of things that I'd spent years not thinking about. Things I'd buried and mistrusted, things I didn't realize I knew. I found a whole attic filled with cobwebs, boxes, and dust. I had no idea what was up there, but I recognized that connecting with my body meant dealing with the attic; traumas, unresolved issues, hurts, habits, and some good memories mixed in. If I were going to move forward, I would have to clear out this space that I'd locked away for 40+ years.

I'd tried going into the attic a few times during the early parts of my recovery, but it was overwhelming. I could tolerate the feelings for only so long and then had to plunge back into numbness, creating an ongoing cycle of binging and restricting.

Once I had God's safety net, though, I could start excavating. I gradually realized that although I thought the attic was shut up tight, I was bringing all that "baggage" into every interaction. Old beliefs, stories, hurts, hangups were coloring and ruining my life experiences. I came to recognize that being overweight was just a symptom of what was going on - and that's true for me now with the toxic mold journey, just as it was before.

I began the work of getting to know the attic and realized there were parts of my psyche that were my guides, but they were stunted and needed healing. They were the ones opening the door, guiding me around, encouraging me to uncover the right things at the right times. It was my job to not leave, shut the door, and tell them to go away. I had to let them take my hand and show me what they wanted me to see.

It was hard as hell and very scary at times. I didn't know how to do what they asked me to do. I was a walking, talking adult child with a very childlike view of the world. My previous hurts were running the show for me, keeping me from my adult mindset.

After the pandemic, I decided to attend a 12-step meeting for dysfunctional families. Seeing how other family dynamics had played out as the individuals grew up and recognizing similarities in my own life was enormously helpful. I began to see that although I felt guilty about the way I had grown, there was actually no other option for me. I could never have turned out any differently than I did because of the experiences I had.

Suddenly, I no longer had to tell the chaperones in my attic that something was wrong with them, that they needed to be hidden, know their place, and keep their mouths shut. They weren't wrong. They were there because they had to be. They had no other choice because of my life experiences. Now, instead of telling parts of myself that they were bad, broken, unworthy, I could accept them.

I also learned I would never get many of the things I was supposed to get from my parents. My mom had died, and her remaining family couldn't give me what I needed. My dad wasn't capable of offering any closure on the wounds he had created. I realized that I was the only one who could do it: no one was coming to save me, nobody else who could fix what was broken. It was on me. I had to do the re-parenting.

I panicked. I'd never had kids. It was a huge loss for me, but I now believe it was for good reason. God had to use the choices that I made for good. He knew that the way I'd adapted to life wouldn't have made me a good parent. I probably would have done major damage to those kids, perhaps recreating the very things I was trying to heal from.

Even so, not having children was still a huge loss, and I was unsure about how to move forward. I had to become my own loving parent, but I had no idea how. My instincts weren't healthy—they were based on fear, scarcity, immaturity, and other behaviors that my family of origin had instilled in me.

I had to quickly find skills that would let me re-parent the damaged parts of myself in healthy ways. Gradually, I got to know all those different parts, different people. I started to learn who they were, what they sounded like, how they behaved, and what they needed and didn't. I saw how they were trying to run my life, navigating situations they had no business navigating. Over time, I figured out how to identify each one and learn how to say, "Thank you, but no thank you; have a seat; I've got this."

Soon, I was able to start a new journey connecting with my true, loving adult self, the person who I really am. It was a very nuanced process, where I found there are 8 parts of my loving adult self, with the most important four being Connected, Compassionate, Curious, and Calm. If I'm not in one of those Cs, I'm in one of my previous parts. I need to slow down, figure out which part of my psyche is running the show, and reclaim control.

Food recovery helped with this, but it also goes many layers deeper. I used to think that if my food was on point and I was exercising, everything else would fall into place, but no. Now, food is a minor aspect of life, just there to provide nourishment. That's as it should be. I have a much deeper connection to myself now than ever before, and it isn't about food or exercise. I can't even exercise much at the moment; I'm supposed to avoid any activity that raises my heart rate until I've started healing.

I now have a lot of time with myself. It would be easy to pick another distraction, zone out, and disconnect from my current physical state, but I don't need to. Doing that makes me resentful, and other parts of my psyche start creeping in and running the show, going back to default settings that take me away from God and recovery.

Instead, I've found a connection to myself, and it involves spending time with my inner family, listening to my body, noticing problematic sensations, and figuring out what's behind them. It involves sharing memories with my inner self, respecting even the parts that I don't want to see, and truly listening. It involves trusting my loving adult self, who can handle anything so that the younger, more damaged parts of my psyche don't feel that it's on them. I'm still sorting through the attic, but much of it has been cleared and dealt with, and in the process, I have uncovered... me.

Paige: Are You Ever Older Than Your First Rejection?

I have heard it said that we are always all the ages that we have ever been. When that concept was first presented to me, I heard it as truth immediately. I recognize that what happened to me in my formative years continues to show up as an adult. Those first cuts still sting when something hits the same spot.

Connection with self is one of the key elements of overcoming food addiction. If you aren't connected with yourself, you don't have the tools to understand what's behind your cravings and emotional eating; you don't have the insight needed to start changing it. You have to get to grips with who you are and what's going on in your head and your heart to reach a point where you can challenge addiction. It's the hardest road you'll ever take, and there's no starting if you don't get to know your passenger (you) before you take the first step.

Addiction is, at its core, seeking to protect us from pain, to numb out the world. It has no understanding of consequences; its sole assignment is to stop pain however it can. To overpower addiction, we've got to get to a place where we can reassure our brains that no, we don't need food; we have other tools that will stop the pain and keep us safe. We can put down the cravings and relax; we can breathe. We're okay. But how do you get to this point?

You have to get to know yourself so you can nurture yourself. I first came across the idea of inner family through Jamie - much later than I would have liked, but what a mind-blowing experience it was.

As an adult, if a love interest ever rejected me, I was instantly brought back to fourth grade when Mike Dehnert shunned my undying devotion and called me ugly (I think he was just mad that I was faster than him in the times tables competition). To be fair, I was a late bloomer in the looks department; he was way out of my league (...at 9), and even then, I understood the natural ranking order when it came to beauty. But the heart still wanted what the heart wanted, and I thought I would never recover from that heartbreak.

As an adult, if I don't get invited to a girl's lunch, I'm right back to hovering wistfully at the edge of the "in crowd" in high school, watching the popular girls band together and wondering what it was that made me the misfit.

And, you're going to love this one: if someone asks to talk to me, my first assumption is that I'm in trouble, and it's my fault. As a hyperactive kid, I got punished a lot, so this one tracks just like the others. There was also the agonizing moment when I was called fat in front of Mr. Huffman's 10th grade English Class by the cutest boy in school.

This is my inner family. I am each of these girls still, decades later. Each one of these injured children lives in my heart, and for years, I never knew that when the wounds were reopened, these kids were the ones who answered the new hurt. I thought it was Adult Me responding to the situations, but no. They were the ones who took control. They governed my reactions and dictated my responses, often in ineffective ways, because, let's face it, they're children. They didn't know that reaching for the cookies wouldn't take the sting out of a rejection.

You've likely experienced this yourself. Moments that hit at our childhood traumas are the moments when we tend to be least proud of how we react. Sometimes, we're baffled by our own responses. Those responses are basically driven by trauma, by an experience that you haven't healed from fully, so it's still following you around and making itself known. By the time you are reading this book, you will have experienced your own set of traumas. Big T traumas or little t traumas, we all have them. Life is just "lifey" that way.

I had plenty, and I realized they were seriously affecting how I operated from day to day, but that didn't help me fix them. So, what am I to do with these insecurities that continue to bubble up? How can I love on those pains, reassure myself that I am safe now, and allow myself to recall events with less trauma, more truth, and greater perspective? How do I train these thinking patterns to rewire themselves into new neural grooves that automatically pull to the positive? I have come to realize that you can curl up in the fetal position or unfurl and develop a relationship with yourself that you can trust.

It took a lot of work for me to reach that point, and I'm still far from perfect. But now, when insecurities pop up, I can ask myself what age that thought is and have a conversation with that little girl. I can picture myself kneeling down with that hurting child, looking her in the eyes, and letting her know she is safe now. I will protect her, and it's all going to be okay. She doesn't have to take the reins because I'm here, and Adult Me is able to take over.

Adult Me can look back at the past with much greater clarity. I now have the ability to process rejection and disappointment. Today, if someone calls me a disparaging name or makes fun of my appearance, I can see that it comes from a damaged place in their own life. Hurt people hurt people. Sadly, as a child, you don't know that.

We all have the ability to talk to our past selves and reassure them that we are safe and have a plan to take care of ourselves. The conversation quiets the addiction, and it was this process that let me get off sugar at long last, with success. In my previous attempts, I'd been led by the children in me, and they weren't ready for it. They weren't going to make a non-negotiable decision and refuse to look back; kids don't have that kind of willpower, confidence, or resilience. They love sweets, and they'll turn to them again and again.

It had to be me, adult Paige, gripping the wheel and holding on tight. I had to tell them, "I got this," and then prove that I had. If I'd never had to face this, I would have never leveled up in my life to become the best version of myself possible: Paige 2.0. I like her a lot because I know her and I trust her. When situations come up that test my recovery, I take that opportunity to remind myself: you have nothing to worry about; I am here and going to keep you safe. You can depend on me. Self-talk really has been one of my biggest allies.

Reconnecting isn't just about boosting your confidence. When you reconnect, you begin to understand the underlying reasons behind cravings and emotional eating. You begin to hear the cues that your body is sending, which sometimes get lost in or stifled by the addiction. You can then find healthier ways to address those needs. Fostering this connection allows you to be more present and make choices that align with your true needs. Ultimately, this journey of reconnection empowers you to take control of your relationship with food and live in a way that supports your overall well-being. It takes patience, self-compassion, and mindfulness, but if you work at it, you can move away from external stimuli and establish a deeper connection with yourself.

That deeper connection helped me in a myriad of ways - not just with food. I have had many opportunities to discover what I am truly made of and become familiar with the deepest parts of myself. I found out I'm pretty cool, and as I like to say, "Alexanders do hard things." While I thought I was just healing my sugar addiction, what really happened is I discovered what my full potential is. I have done things I never thought I could do, I have helped others do what they never thought they could do, and I have created things I never thought I could create. In many ways, my addiction has helped me because it forced me to get in touch with myself and figure out how to take the wheel.

The RFR Takeaways

How To Connect With Yourself

Connecting with yourself on a deep level takes more tools than we can possibly cover in this book, and for many people, it will involve engaging with communities and professionals so that they can gain the techniques needed for this. However, there are some elements we can introduce you to here that will start the journey for you.

Confidence-Building

Find activities that elevate your confidence and belief in your own ability to handle things. That might involve taking on stretch projects at work, doing some courses to expand your skills, or working with a therapist or other professional who can help you see the value you bring to the world. Often, when we do the things we're afraid of, we build our confidence, but you do have to set yourself up to succeed. Find things that challenge you but don't overwhelm you, and do thorough preparation. Get others involved to help you. Look for opportunities that push your boundaries but not too much.

This kind of thing can massively boost your sense of self and your willingness to step up to challenges and take on difficulties. It will help in all different areas - not just the one where you're specifically focusing on growth. Becoming aware of our self-talk, another branch of the tree, can help us become more emotionally intelligent, heal some of those inner wounds, and regain control over our lives.

Reframing

Reframing is a powerful technique that changes how you look at things. When something happens, we each build it into a narrative about how things are going and what's likely to come next. Looking at things neutrally is hard, and many of us end up with a negative lens that is not constructive.

Reframing involves changing the lens and finding the positive, even in a negative situation. It's what gets you through when disappointment comes knocking. It lets you look at the bigger picture and take into account the idea that this bad thing might ultimately lead somewhere good.

Take a moment to look back over your life and think about how things that seemed terrible on the surface eventually did take you through to something positive. Perhaps a breakup led to you meeting your long-term partner, or getting laid off led you to a better job. Many of us jump to the worst possible conclusion, undermining ourselves and our ability to handle the challenges of life.

When this happens, work on mentally reframing so that you can meet challenges with an open mind and a willingness to see the positives as well as the negatives. You'll find obstacles and setbacks far less stressful if you can achieve this.

Mindfulness

Learning how to be more mindful takes time, but it's worth the effort. You'll hear this talked about a lot, and essentially, it means taking some time to be in the present moment every day: feeling the sensations of your body, listening to your thoughts, and accepting your emotions as they exist.

It's about paying attention to just existing in that moment, listening to the sensations, and feeling yourself in the world. You can be mindful while chopping vegetables for dinner while sitting on the bus traveling home or for 10 minutes before you go to bed. If you can create a habit of mindfulness, you'll find yourself more in tune with your body and its sensations and better capable of managing your inner family. They will all feel heard and understood, meaning they're less likely to start shouting when a crisis hits.

Get Informed

Spend a bit of time thinking specifically about your inner family and what you think the dominant forces of your psyche are. Consider what your biggest pain points in life have been and where these might be causing weaknesses or further friction. Think about - or better yet, write about - the things you dislike in yourself, and then spend a bit of time sitting with these things, ruminating on how they affect you, what benefits they bring, and what you can do to give them less control in your life.

Remember that knowledge is power: the better you know your weaknesses and strengths, the better you can limit and utilize them. It takes time to identify these things in yourself, but it's worth the effort, and you can get assistance from loved ones if you need it.

Be Alone

Although loneliness is not good for our mental health, it's important to know how to be by yourself and to feel comfortable with this. Being alone gives your thoughts room, lets your brain breathe, and allows more scope for mindfulness. Try to make some space that is just yours from time to time, whether that involves taking a long bath, sitting in a room on your own, going for a solitary walk, or something else. Embrace moments when you are alone and learn to enjoy your own company. It's something that many of us struggle with, especially when grappling with food issues, but it will grant you a lot of insight and often a sense of peace and comfort that can't be achieved through other means.

Hopefully, those will set your feet on the right path to undertake this journey. Reach out your hand and greet yourself: you are now starting a connection that will serve you for a lifetime. In the next chapter, we will look at relationships with others, another crucial facet of staying on the lifeboat, keeping yourself afloat, and putting food into the right place in your life.

CHAPTER 8

Connection To Others

For many people, the quality of their relationships with others is the biggest determining factor in their happiness. That's not to say that we should seek to get all our fulfillment from others or that others should dictate how happy we feel. It's just saying that as a social species, we can make ourselves happier when we enjoy genuine, healthy, balanced relationships with the people around us.

Here at RFR, we often say community is the antidote for addiction. That's what makes it a key branch of our program. Being on the lifeboat with other people is one of the best ways to make sure you stay on the boat, for a whole host of reasons. It's partly that seeing others there gives you the confidence that you can be there, too. It's partly that nobody wants to be stuck on a lifeboat all by themselves. It's partly that others can give you advice about navigating the seas, tips on the monsters to avoid, and maybe even a helping hand to keep you aboard when the sea is choppy. Humans are wired for connection and we need others around us if we're going to succeed.

That's true even for introverts who often prefer to "go it alone." We still depend on our support networks when times are tough, and we still find joy and fulfillment in helping each other through difficult patches.

Perhaps most importantly, community helps us to come out of ourselves and be part of something bigger, whereas addiction tends to be an isolating, self-centered experience. When you're connected with others, you're less likely to be focused on just eating; you're less likely to hear the sound of addiction. You have other things keeping you happy and bringing you a sense of safety, reducing the need to eat.

We know that loneliness breeds addiction, and it stands to reason that satisfying your instinctive need for companionship reduces your risk of going overboard and into the water. So, let's look at connectedness to others.

Jamie: Boundaries and Detachment

I've discussed the importance of community throughout this book, but in this chapter, I want to take a different approach and examine the importance of connecting specifically in healthy ways —and, by extension, disconnecting or at least distancing when necessary.

During my recovery, I found that as we heal, our relationships change. It wasn't just in terms of the people I used food with, but other relationships, too. I had to alter how I spent time with people, find different things to do, and learn to say "no" when invited to a restaurant or cafe. That was hard, but necessary. I'd spent most of my life building relationships that revolved around food: eating out, going over for dinner, checking out unique food opportunities like fairs or street stalls. There were certainly other activities, too, but food was the focus.

I had to learn how to change my focus. It started with figuring out how to speak up for my needs and working out how to compromise. Often, since I was married, it wasn't just about what I wanted to do, but what he wanted - meaning I didn't feel like I could give a straight "no" every time. I started to bring my own food and approach the activity differently, but it caused a lot of problems.

People felt I was not the same person, that I was uptight, perhaps even that I was judging them. I internalized much of that feedback for a long time. I felt ashamed, judged, and frustrated with myself even though I was beginning an important, health-critical journey. Sometimes, I thought maybe I should give up and go back to old habits to keep the peace. I had to remind myself that I was saving my life. I couldn't give in to what was essentially peer pressure. I had to put myself first.

It was hard. Sometimes, I could say "yes" to an invitation if it was after the meal, or I could suggest non-food activities, but not always. Some people stopped wanting to spend time with me. Relationships changed; relationships ended. It was immensely painful at points; I lost some people I loved deeply, people I'd shared good connections and fun memories with - not all food-related. Over time, I realized that I was being pruned; God was cutting away unhealthy or damaging connections to give me space to grow. I hated losing those people, hated being rejected for standing up for my needs, and at points, I doubted myself... but I kept going. Some people were in my life for reasons and seasons, while others were there for the long haul.

I had to put in more effort, preserving the parts of the friendship that mattered while I stripped away parts that didn't. On the flip side, I had to learn how to care for myself in relationships that weren't good for me. Some were unhealthy and dysfunctional, and the more I healed, the more I could see it. I had to walk away. Those relationships were not life-giving; they were anxiety-producing or dysfunctional. I needed to trust myself and my feelings; if my heart felt full, the relationship was serving me. If I didn't feel emotionally safe - no matter how much I liked the person - I needed to listen and step away.

I knew I was doing the right thing, and I knew nobody else was going to take on this fight. Over time, the feelings of shame and judgment became an exercise in creating boundaries. At the start, I was clumsy, struggling to say no in ways that protected the relationship. I was sometimes too fierce and failed to take the other person's feelings into consideration or spent too much time explaining and getting bogged down in my words. The biggest lesson was that "no" is a complete sentence. I didn't have to defend my choices or give a long explanation. That was just trying to squelch my guilt/indecision.

Gradually, I mastered the art of boundary-setting in ways that took care of me and protected the other person. I learned and made mistakes. The people who were good for me understood and forgave me. Others who were not healthy would often perpetuate the issue or guilt-trip me. That was helpful because it let me see that I felt constantly worse being around them, and they weren't my people. They weren't out to get me, and I wasn't a victim. It was just that my unhealed parts were triggering their unhealed parts and contributing to dysfunction. In some cases, where healing has been done on both sides, we're still friends and we can share much more functional relationships. It took time, but we got there.

Unfortunately, this process of boundary-setting also came with self-judgment and condemnation. I wondered if I was being a fair-weather friend. I had to remind myself that I had a bigger goal and my health - not just my food, but my overall health - was more important. Dysfunctional relationships affected it. I had to be honest about which relationships were good and which weren't so I could reach my goals. I also had to figure out how to take the relationships that could be preserved and make them better for both parties.

Here, I want to talk about the tool of "detachment." There are many different ways to detach. You can detach from your emotions, their emotions, negative thoughts, outcomes to situations, assumptions, and much more. As I worked on my relationships, I spent a lot of time practicing non-attachment and it became a critical tool. When I was attached, I was along for whatever ride they chose to take me on. I was very co-dependent. My moods and outlooks reflected theirs. I was basing my perceptions on others. It was a roller-coaster and not a pleasant one. It left me with little understanding of who I was, what I wanted, what I thought, or what was good for me. I put too much into people-pleasing and changing myself to meet someone else's expectations.

So it was time for boundaries, with a detached mindset. Interestingly, I learned that boundaries involve other people, but detachment is a decision that belongs to you alone. Others don't have to know about it; they don't get a say. When you detach, you recognize where you end and where others begin, and you can reassign their feelings to them. These things are not your business, because you aren't looking at the world through the same lens. You can't see what they see, no matter how you try; let go and focus on the world in front of you. Feel your feelings and acknowledge your perceptions.

It's not easy for most of us to do that. I'm very empathetic, so I take on people being disappointed, sad, happy, or mad, and I want to fix it. That's the definition of co-dependence. Now, I realize I was not put on this Earth to fix other human beings. I had to detach from their emotions and from the stories in my head about what they were thinking or what the outcomes would be. I had to let it go. Nobody knew I was doing it, but I did it for me.

Boundaries and detachment go well together in relationships. They helped me keep myself safe in recovery and also stay as emotionally healthy and emotionally available as I could be.

Here's an example of what this looked like for me: I had a relationship with a close friend who was always very supportive and present in my life. I turned to her for advice, approval, insight, input on everything. Because I had a lot of unhealed stuff, I became very enmeshed with her, constantly seeking her feedback. Unfortunately, I was so unhealed that I couldn't see the issue of co-dependence. I began to base my sense of worth on her opinions. It put me in a situation where I was subject to her judgments, and naturally, those weren't always positive. She was also a big part of my network, so those judgments impacted how others saw me too. It was very hurtful and damaging to my self-esteem.

I had to figure out how I could keep this person in my life but change the dynamic. Her good qualities far outweighed her bad ones, and I couldn't have borne losing her. I was beginning to heal myself, and I knew that my friend would never intentionally hurt anyone she loved... yet somehow I was always getting hurt, and I couldn't figure out why.

When I began my recovery journey, I thought that if you were close to someone, they had to have full access to you at all times. You had to tell them everything. It's not true.

When I came across the concept of concentric circles as a means of understanding relationships, it blew my mind. Your innermost circles are for the most important people, while the outer circles are for those who are less connected. People can move around depending on the circumstances and the needs of the relationship.

At the start of my recovery, this person was in my bullseye, a place now occupied by only myself and God. She knew all my inner thoughts and fears. Having her so close was not healthy for us, because my unhealed things were triggering her unhealed things. I had to learn how to move her, with love and care, from my bullseye to an outer circle. I had to preserve the relationship and honor the love and history, but set healthy boundaries.

I practiced detachment from her judgment and her attempts to help me, which were very dysfunctional for both of us. It took time, and I had to get some distance, both physically and emotionally. I had to be mindful of what I shared and figure out what I could limit. I had to protect both of us throughout the process. It was a lot of work, but we're now in a place where we enjoy a healthy, balanced friendship that is well-kept, nurtured, and far more functional than before.

I love my friend's humanity, her history, her connection. She's like a sister to me still, but she does not dictate my sense of self-worth. She doesn't dictate who I am, what I do, or what matters. I am my own person, at the center of my bullseye, and I assign others to the circles around me in ways that are healthy.

Through this process, I've figured out how to build connections that nourish me, keep me on the lifeboat, and retain my balance. Community, as you will have realized in the other chapters, is critical to my functioning, but it has to be right, and you have to preserve your sense of self as you interact with others.

Paige: The Shadow Behind Me

Connection to others is a subject I sometimes find hard to write about because I'm a self-described loner. I don't have, or want, a huge network of friends to go out to brunch with; I'm not into shopping trips or hours-long phone calls with my bestie. And yet, for me, connection is still an invaluable part of getting through life, clean eating, and mental health.

It was again during my husband's battle with sepsis that this was brought home to me most clearly. During the second or third week, when I was getting to the hospital at 7 a.m. every morning so I could talk to the doctors eyeball-to-eyeball (see, there's an instance where connection was really serving me), I had one moment that was particularly poignant.

I was in the elevator, lost in thought, wondering what I would find upstairs, what this day would bring. I was praying for just another day with my husband. I pushed the button marked "3" and, without realizing it, let out a huge sigh. The weight of the world was in that sigh, and from behind me came a quiet voice. "Me too."

I looked around and found a man standing behind me, unnoticed in the shadows. Our eyes met, and we shared a split-second connection, one of the most profound in my life. This human and I were living the same reality. We were walking in the same shoes. Nobody understood us better than the other. Standing in a metal box full of raw emotion, two strangers trauma bonding across just a few moments, reassuring each other without words that we were not alone in our struggles. We were understood. We were seen. Our sighs were heard and recognized for their depth.

He got off at Floor 2, heading to face whatever the universe had in store for him and his loved one that day. I went up one more floor. I never saw him again. And yet he gave me a precious gift: a moment to turn the focus away from my suffering and say a prayer for all those who were hurting in the universe. We were all in this together; our cumulative pain linked us. Those few seconds of connectedness gave me the strength to get through that day, and many others. I will never forget that man. I have no idea what his name was or what his trials were, but I know that we stood together as warriors in the face of great pain, and that will stay with me always.

This is connection for me. I find it in many other - less stressful - situations, too. Interestingly, I feel most connected to people who I see on a daily basis, even if I don't have a clue what their names are or what other parts of their lives are like. They connect with me in fundamental ways. The people I see at the gym before sunrise every morning - the man in the purple shirt, the lady in her Lulus, the guy sporting WSU gear (Go Shocks), and the trainer who is always smiling. I don't know these people, but I know them. They are my people, and we share that experience of early morning exercise. I know I'll leave every interaction energized, not drained. They are all examples of who I want to be and how I want to start each day. The fire in their bellies is contagious. They are living my priorities and it's enormously motivating.

I feel a deep sense of connection to every head nod and "good morning," and I know that I will feel good every time I show up. Starting with this foundation, surrounded by my nameless tribe, makes every day better. We connect not through words but through lived experiences.

It's not just at the gym; I thrive in the familiarity of seeing the same people at the same places everywhere. The people at the grocery store, the families sitting on their same pews in church - even my workmates. These are stable influences in the life of a lady who hates change (and that's an understatement). I find these consistent forces lightly touching me as I go throughout my day, and I love it. It is emotional stability for me (It is not lost on me that there is no expectation on my part). Ironically, they don't even know I depend on them to show up to make sure my world continues to spin on its axis.

For example, I've had the same Santa Claus come to our house at 5 p.m. on Christmas Eve for the last 30 years, a tradition that started when my husband and I were first dating, with our combined family of 5 kids aged 2-13. Now, those children's children sit on Santa's lap. He appears in every photo album we own. This is connection to me (Santa, you complete me). These are the people who fill my lifeboat.

These thoughts leave me wondering: Am I silently important to others? Have they connected themselves to me? Would Santa even recognize Christmas if he didn't come to my house? Have I imprinted on his holiday traditions?

You never know what impact you leave on others, as our oldest twin granddaughter reminded me the other day. We were chatting in my daughter's kitchen, and she said, "Glamma, why do you always try to look pretty?"

I looked at her, perplexed, so she continued, "You know, your hair always looks like this-" waving her hand in the air, drawing a half circle mirroring the back of my head "-and you always wear lipstick."

I took a few minutes to explain the definition of vain, and thought about how my own mother had always told me and my two younger sisters to never leave the house without lipstick. "You look dead without it," she'd say. Spruce up, tease the back of your crown for volume; it puts you at an advantage in the world. I asked her recently where it all came from, assuming the lipstick tradition was passed down from her mother, that there was a deep-rooted connection that had linked generations of our women over the importance of always looking your best.

Surprisingly, it hadn't come from her mother, and she said she didn't know, beyond, "Basically, you three were just pale." Well, she wasn't wrong. But guess what I have done all my adult life when I first get out of bed? Put on my lipstick... I refuse to look dead.

So when I stop and think about what makes a relationship worthwhile to me - what motivates me to move out of my loner habits long enough to pick up the phone and send a text or funny cat video - I have to conclude that I do it to feel good, warm on the inside, part of something bigger, as though I have a purpose. I want to be connected to the universe on a deeper level. I want to connect with people who bring out the best version of myself. I want to know I mean something to them, too.

And I know that I want to have boundaries where necessary, a concept I hadn't even understood until my mid-50s. I know that over the years, I accepted a lot of treatment that I should not have permitted (by the way, that's on me, not them). I have come to know that if boundaries are not enforced, they are nothing more than a simple request. I needed to develop the self-esteem and self-confidence to stand up for myself and be willing to walk away if I wasn't being treated as I deserved.

I know how easy it is to blur them when it comes to family and long-term friendships, and that's one reason I was grateful to Jamie for introducing me to the idea of concentric circles. Here, the bullseye is the command post that houses your most intimate and trustworthy relationships. When people don't meet the criteria for that one, you can move them to an outer circle without having to cut all ties. This lets you be safe while still maintaining some contact. We're keeping the metaphorical baby while getting rid of the bathwater. It's not right for every situation, but it helped me a lot. It meant I didn't have to choose all or nothing when somebody was damaging my life; I could assign them to a space that was right for my needs in that moment. Navigating tricky relationships while in recovery is vital to maintaining abstinence, because stress from relationships can be highly triggering.

So, what is it about connection that matters to me? Some think that time spent together is what defines a good relationship - others put it down to blood relationships, to school friendships, or to excellent working partnerships. For me, it's about shared experiences and quality over quantity. My two best girlfriends are my daughters. A lot of time is spent texting and calling. In-person time can be a luxury when life is busy and you're raising families. As adults, everything we do and every move we make has a payoff, or we wouldn't do it. So what am I looking for when it comes to connection, what's the payoff?

I know I'm "choosy" about who I spend time with and how we spend it. If I like you, I'll invite you to come hiking, work out, play tennis, or meet me at the zoo with the grandkids. I want to share air space with those who have like-minded goals and values. Time is precious, and I want to grow when I interact. I joined my hiking group because I wanted to join in with the activity, and as a payoff, I've been to places I'd never have gone alone, and had experiences I could never have imagined. I thrive when spending time with people who go to bed early, prioritize health, and share my faith. These connections reinforce my beliefs and make me feel part of something bigger than myself.

My last half marathon held great significance for me—though at the time, I had no idea it would be my last. My goal was to beat my personal record of 2 hours and 10 minutes, and I did—by exactly one second. (I'm counting it!) This was the coveted Rock 'n' Roll Half Marathon, run at night along the infamous Las Vegas Strip. The bright city lights illuminated our roped-off course, but what I didn't expect were the throngs of people lining the streets for miles, hands outstretched for "side high-fives" as we ran past. I had never experienced anything like it in any other race. The energy was electric. Every single touch sent a jolt of power through me, pushing me forward. Connection raced through my veins. #PunIntended. My inner drive to be a great runner was reignited. It was a high like no other—the crowd loved me, and I was eating it up.

But then, the Strip's neon glow faded. The crowds thinned, then vanished. The final miles were lit only by dim streetlights, and I was left with nothing but my own effort to carry me through. The other runners around me weren't cheering me on or showing me any love; they were simply surviving their own race. My moment of fame had passed, and with it, the illusion of deep connection. I realized then: what I had experienced was nothing more than a fleeting, surface-level interaction—energizing, yes, but ultimately shallow. That kind of support, built on convenience and spectacle, isn't sustainable. It isn't real.

As I have aged, I truly have come to value the connections I have with the few like-minded people I cherish spending time with, and the boost I get from experience-sharing with the strangers in my world. And if it's true that obesity is contagious, it seems that a healthy lifestyle could be too - so I spend my time connecting with people that share my core beliefs: single-ingredient food, sleep, movement, and spirituality. While my connections may be few in numbers, they are great in significance.

The RFR Takeaways

Building Connections

Let's say it bluntly: connections are a lot of work. We have to set boundaries. We have to manage feelings, and we have to figure out healthy, productive, and beneficial ways to interact. It takes effort and many of us get it wrong at times. Even so, connections are - as we said at the start of this chapter - critical to recovery. Whether we like it or not, we're part of a giant network of people, and we have to interact with each other to function.

Community helps us fight addiction because it fulfills us. We are naturally social creatures and we don't do well with isolation. Addiction often seeks to isolate us, because of the shame and guilt attached to it, which is why it's even more critical to deliberately seek connections and create empathetic, trusting, nurturing networks that will let us thrive. This lifeboat isn't you on your own; we're here too, as are thousands of others! Seeing that can, in itself, help. So, how do we propose building connections?

Use Concentric Circles

Both of us mentioned concentric circles in our personal journeys, and it's because they are so immensely valuable. These circles help us to get into a state of constantly assessing our relationships and determining how well they are serving us - or not - in the given context. We can then move people closer or shift them further away depending on our current needs. We can also respect other people's circles and recognize that our position in these is likely to fluctuate as contexts and needs change.

You will also become more deliberate about what you do and don't share and find it easier to detach from other people's emotions because they will become self-contained entities in your mind. They won't bleed into your sense of self so easily. Furthermore, it can make it easier to step back when you need to because you can move somebody to one of your outer circles without having to make the hard decision to cut them out of your life entirely.

Find Your People

We all thrive on different things in life; finding people you connect with makes all the difference. Many of us bond through shared activities or experiences, so look for things you love doing, and find people through that. Whether it's exercise, art, music, literature, education, or any of the other myriad of activities, find your people. Look for ones who make you feel good, who fill your cup instead of emptying it, and trust your instincts. Remember, we reflect those around us, so we want to be surrounded by positive, growth-focused individuals.

Think About Food's Functionality In The Relationship

Many of us bond around food; it's a big part of life for vast swathes of society. It's embedded in our cultures and traditions. All our huge events tend to focus on it. Whether it's Thanksgiving or Christmas at home, a work celebratory dinner, a birthday meal out with friends... food is pretty much a given at some time or another in most of your relationships. Of course, you can consciously reduce that, but even so, there's likely to be some intersection, so use that to gain insight into how the relationship works.

Is the person respectful of your choices and supportive of your needs? Do they listen when you say "no"? Do they avoid stepping over your boundaries? This often tells you what the relationship is like overall! If they're pressuring you to eat things that you don't want, ignoring your preferences, or goading you, they're likely disrespecting you in other ways, too. If they are neutral or supportive, it's probably a healthier, more functional relationship!

Our relationships tend to affect our food choices in very fundamental ways. When you feel fulfilled, heard, and respected by those around you, you don't look at food to fill that hole. You don't "need" it in that way anymore. Equally, when you don't put food at the core of everything, you can focus on your relationships and find far more joy and fulfillment in the wonderful people around you - not in eating. Your connections will get deeper, stronger, and richer because you're paying attention to the other person.

Indeed, this is partly why we depend on food in so many social situations; it smooths the interactions and reduces the intensity of our focus on each other. When you take away the food, things can get more awkward... or far more rewarding. Your relationships will certainly change when you take food out of the equation, but almost always for the better.

Approach With Patience

Patience will be one of your greatest tools on this journey, and it applies to yourself and others. We often forget just how valuable patience is, and in a world that's jam-packed, it can be easy to feel irritated when it seems your time is being wasted, but ultimately, patience and forgiveness will serve you when it comes to connecting with both yourself and others.

Starting with self, patience will help you in a multitude of ways, especially when you slip up and miss a goal. Remind yourself that this isn't about perfection, and nobody's expecting to see an instant, overnight change. You haven't failed. You haven't wasted all your hard work. You're not back at square one. Cut the negative thoughts and recognize that this is a step back, not a restart.

Next, your relationships. This is a big change, and none of us like change! Some people will be shocked, and even good friends may not initially be as supportive as we would like. They might let you down. Be patient with them and recognize that if they are good people, they will support you. As you expect some grace in your moments of imperfection, give some grace in other people's moments. It will make life a lot easier for everyone.

That doesn't mean you have to let people trample all over your boundaries; it just means not getting hung up on the little things, and giving time for people to adjust. Treat those around you with kindness, even if you ultimately decide to detach, because it will make the journey better for everyone - you included.

Having a good community around you is one of the most powerful ways you can fight addiction and get on the path to recovery, not to mention stay there. They'll keep you in this lifeboat we're all striving to stay aboard. Joining the RFR community is a great way to find people who know exactly what you're going through, but look in your local area and in your hobbies, too. Connections are crucial, and with the right tools, you can build ones that will serve you for a lifetime.

In the next chapter, we're going to start looking at mindset and how it can help you gather your resilience for the journey that lies ahead. Our lifeboat is almost fully equipped with the major tools needed for recovery; let's plunge into the next topic!

CHAPTER 9

Mindset

Who is going on this food journey with you? Maybe your partner, your kids, your friends? Ultimately, this comes down to you and your brain. It's going to be the two of you battling it out for control of what goes into your mouth, and if your brain isn't on board, you're not really on the lifeboat yet. You've got to find a mindset that will keep you aboard even when the seas are rough, and that's what this chapter is going to help with.

What we think about a situation is far more powerful than many of us realize. The way we approach things sets us up for success or failure in some very major ways. Most of us believe we interact with the "true" version of reality, that we are focused only on what's real but actually, that's kind of impossible. We interact with reality filtered through all our lenses, preconceptions, emotions, beliefs, hangups, perspectives, and more. We constantly interpret the world and then react to that interpretation rather than what's actually happening. Part of this involves your personal values and following your purpose in life, two more branches on our tree.

What that means is that your mindset is one of the most important tools. If you believe you're capable of doing this, you'll be in for a much easier time than if your mind is constantly sabotaging you with doubts. Your mind can set you free - but you've got to believe in yourself. If you're wobbly in your brain, you are really just making life harder; if you set a rule and stick to it, everything becomes easy. The rule of "no negotiation" is easier to stick to than "negotiate sometimes." We're going to cover the power of mindset and some techniques you can use later on in the chapter, but first, let us talk a bit about what mindset means to us.

Jamie: What Do You Do With Lemons?

My mindset has evolved a lot as I've grown into an adult. Many of the people in my early life taught me about the victim mindset. They had an outlook that sought to blame the external world. Everything was being done "at" them. Someone else was always at fault when things went wrong. I thought that was how everybody looked at life.

All problems had to be passed to somebody else. It was an enormously disempowering environment because when you blame others for things that happen to you, you give them the power over the situation. You put your life and feelings in their hands. It causes enormous amounts of stress, resentment, and animosity because we're giving away our control and letting others dictate how we think and feel. That's just how I thought the world worked. None of us were empowered; we drifted along, trying to minimize the hurt that others did to us.

It was a terrible place to be. I was constantly at odds with the world, always afraid, and always looking for people to blame. I had no idea there were alternative mindsets that you could adopt. My young experiences taught me that when life gives you lemons, you've got to squirt them in somebody else's face. Until I was in my 30s, I had never heard of making lemonade.

My mother, in particular, modeled negative approaches. She deeply believed other people were out to hurt us, and we had to carry around grudges. It was how she dealt with hurt when it came in: hold on tight and burn your hands rather than putting it down. My parents divorced when I was about seven, and my mother never let go of her grudge against my dad and his choices. She clung to her anger and resentment like they would keep her head above water.

It affected her health and all her choices. It stopped her from going after things, and it hindered her future relationships. She was the victim, and she was never going to forget it. They say that holding onto resentment is like drinking poison and expecting somebody else to die, and that was very much what I saw in her. She only hurt herself.

And when she died very young, there was no doubt that her health had been compromised because she clung to that bitterness for so long. She had abused food, grown addicted to chemicals, preservatives, calories, and unhealthy ingredients, and destroyed her body to the point that she couldn't fight off the infections she kept picking up from the kids at her school. It was a miserable place for her to be, and it was all because she couldn't put the lemons down.

The grief was very deep for all of us; she was at the core of our family, and everybody loved her. To lose her so suddenly was painful in ways that are hard to describe. I'll never forget what happened after her funeral, though. My uncle-in-law, who was like a brother to my mom, approached me.

"If you don't think that your mom's anger and the grudge she held toward your dad contributed to her death, you're wrong. I'm telling you this because I don't want you to ever hold onto anything that deep for that long because it will affect your health. I need you to understand that your mother died an early death because she couldn't let these things go."

I didn't really understand what he meant. I was a positive, sunny person, I thought. My glass was half full. I agreed with the sentiments, but until I had my own difficult life experiences, I didn't grasp what he was talking about, and I had no idea my mindset was exactly the same as hers. After all, nobody had ever taught me you could choose differently! It took another decade before I understood that I could, in fact, choose.

I carried that lack of understanding with me throughout my young adulthood, both before and after my mom died. I believed that people either made me better or dragged me down; I had no control, and I felt like I had to be immensely selective about who I spent time with. I tried to control everything I could, even other people, although I didn't realize it at the time. I was just trying to keep myself from getting hurt.

The approach left me both stressed and afraid. I didn't go out of my comfort zone; I didn't look for ways to speak up, assert myself, or ask for opportunities. Part of it was because of my lack of faith in God, who had been shown to me as a fearful overlord who judged and punished. I wouldn't put my faith in Him because I believed He was out to hurt me, too. I set myself against the whole world. I thought I had to have a death grip on life if I had any chance of surviving. What a way to live.

I spent my 20s and some of my early 30s like that, with slow shifts starting when I saw the way others interacted with the world. People who looked for the good, who didn't hold onto blame, and who were unafraid interested me. I had many different informal tutors, including the coaches and therapists I worked with in my 30s as I was going through my divorce. I gradually realized that although I thought I was generally optimistic, I was actually living in a place of victimhood, where I believed that I had done bad things to others and that others had done bad things to me. There was no forgiveness either for me or them. There was no scope for second chances.

Watching others helped me change that, as did my return to spirituality. Some people stand out as particularly influential, with my father-in-law being one. I remember an incident where he was the victim of fraud and lost thousands of dollars. It had an enormous impact on his life, with all the stress of getting it sorted out, but what I really remember about the situation is how calm he was. He told me about it, and when he walked away, he was whistling. I remember feeling baffled. How could he do that? How could he feel so light when somebody had targeted him in such an awful way?

I asked him about it later, questioning how he could let stuff go and sleep at night. He smiled and said, "I sleep great. It's not up to me. God's got it."

I never heard him get angry because when life gave him lemons, he either made lemonade or put the lemons down and walked away. They didn't affect him. And he passed that ethos on to my husband in ways that I will forever admire and cherish. He's been a mentor to me, too, guiding my thoughts and helping me to change my perspective.

Two other friends have also helped me to look at things the way that God would want me to. They've helped me get to grips with the idea of mindset and the purpose of having faith, even if I can't understand what's happening or I feel like it doesn't make sense. I have to be able to say, "Okay, I don't get it and I'm angry, but I trust God and I want Him to help me look at this differently until I feel better or something changes."

That approach has helped me enormously; during my 30s and 40s, I saw some truly incredible evolution. I'm not perfect, but I now know that I can choose to adopt a different mindset and change my feelings. I can't control others, but I can forgive them and move forward. My faith in God has really helped with this. I know He wants what's right for me, so I'm not in a place of fear the way I used to be.

That was really put to the test when I recently hit more health difficulties, and my body started struggling. I felt like I was being put through the wringer, and the road ahead seemed impossibly long. It took me some time to realize that while I couldn't change being sick, I could change how I felt. I wasn't healing as fast as I wanted, but I could still choose to feel good. I could still look at the best elements of my life. I believe that God would want me to choose a positive mindset and put my faith in Him and His guidance rather than worrying about the minutiae.

Once I started reminding myself that I could choose to feel happiness, contentment, hope, and faith, everything became easier. I put down the sadness, resentment, and anger and worked on accepting where I am. I still hope that things will get better, but just being okay with the now marks such a peaceful, helpful shift. I got my lessons late in life, but I'm certainly using them, and the difference to how I feel is indescribable.

Paige: The Mental Muscle Determines Success

Before Covid hit, I would regularly go into the studios of our local ABC affiliate, KAKE TV, and do live cooking presentations on air. Once the world shut down, the station couldn't allow guests in the studio and I had to start pre-recording at home and send them in. One of the segments I filmed was centered around kids, so I had my twin granddaughters record that one with me. I had the perfect setup in my kitchen with lights, a camera and plenty of action. At the end of the recording, I told the girls to wave goodbye to the imaginary audience, which they did with great animation.

But as soon as I pushed stop and the cameras went down, one of the girls said, "Glamma, who is the audience?"

It struck me that it is hard to understand the things we cannot see. Waving goodbye to an invisible crowd doesn't make sense when there's no basis for understanding. Equally, it's hard to stop eating Doritos when we can't see directly into our mitochondria that are begging for mercy. If we haven't been hit by heart disease, diabetes, or cancer, then everything must be okay, right? Since we don't have a telescope to our internal organs, it often takes a huge mental push to break a habit before problems arise, even if logic tells us we need to make changes.

During Nursing School, we learned in our Mental Health semester that people typically only make a change during a crisis; otherwise, most lack the motivation even if change would do them good. Why is that? Well, for humans, part of protecting our existence involves trying to conserve energy wherever possible, and that includes within our thoughts. It's easier to be lazy in the brain and feel satisfied with mediocrity than to challenge ourselves. That rut can seem very comfortable, especially because any change can be detected as danger. It's the devil we know, and one I am personally familiar with.

That's the first observation I wanted to make about mindset. We don't like to change. Our mental muscle is comfortable where it is, and prefers inertia. Hurdle one is often figuring out how to overcome that inertia and get yourself moving.

Onto the second observation!

During the 2024 Summer Paris Olympics, I watched a gymnast competing on the balance beam. She fell off after an in-air stunt and landed on the mat with a thud. The announcer immediately said it was obvious what happened (maybe to him). "She was looking at the ground."

My takeaway was that your focus determines your trajectory. In simpler terms, your energy flows where your focus goes. When I was learning to play tennis, my instructor repeatedly shouted, "Don't take your eye off the ball. " Whenever I hit a bad shot, his broken-record self would repeat, "Well, you took your eye off the ball, didn't you?"

An eye roll response typically represented my sophomoric contrition... but although I would never admit it to him, it was a huge lesson in how powerful our thoughts are. To say they change outcomes and determine our future would be an understatement. Our mental game is an essential part of scoring points.

Mindset plays a crucial role in overcoming the effects of ultra-processed food addiction because it shapes how people approach challenges, setbacks, and ultimately, their recovery. A positive mindset helps individuals shift from feeling powerless against cravings to feeling empowered to make healthier choices. You might think of it as an abundant mindset versus an abstinent mindset. It's literally a matter of perspective, and we get to choose how we think about things.

When I had my first success with refraining from sugar during a family event, it changed my world. I did a lot of preparation beforehand; my head was in the game, and success was non-negotiable. The only thing that got me through that first win was what was happening between my ears. Then, after that experience, I had the knowledge that I could do it. It was a first. It wasn't easy, but I realized I had way more power than I had ever given myself credit for. It changed my life. And it started with attitude and desire. When someone believes they can control their actions, they're more likely to succeed. You have to cultivate the belief that you have the power to make healthy choices and overcome temptations.

Was I 100% successful from that day forward? No, definitely not. There were setbacks from time to time, but my thinking around those changed, too. I could beat myself up or make a decision that my shortcomings were nothing more than lessons to be learned - growth opportunities if you will. Those thoughts can then lead into loving and understanding versus beating ourselves up. Being negative puts you in dangerous territory and makes you far more likely to give up. And I only have one rule when it comes to recovering from the effects of ultra-processed, chemically-engineered foods... never give up. That's your only job.

I also learned that our future selves play a big role in staying the course. Oftentimes, at night, irrational hunger sets in, and that's when most people feel wobbly. Just the other day, I overheard a couple of older gentlemen talking at the gym, and one was saying, "I eat so healthy during the day, but I bet I eat 1,000 calories of ice cream at night. I just can't help it." Patting his stomach, he continued, "I bet I could lose this belly if I could change that habit."

I would love nothing more than to go to his house every night and join him in his ice cream binge, but my future self would not be pleased when I woke up the next morning (and my husband might have questions as well). One of the biggest things that has helped me in getting my mind on board with my goals is hyper focusing on how good I will feel when I am successful. I can't count the number of times that's changed my inner dialogue from "I can't do this" to "I am going to be so happy when I wake up clean in the morning." And every morning when I wake up successful, I always remember to thank myself for taking such good care of me. Self-trust shapes self-talk because it reduces fear of failure and encourages persistence. It is a direct path to inner peace and calm.

This is again about changing your perspective and your focus. Sometimes, we get caught up in dwelling on what we're giving up rather than what we're gaining. Our focus should be on having an abundant mindset, but too often, we focus on the loss instead. I have had people question if I am really not going to have cookies at Christmas, pie at Thanksgiving, or candy at Halloween ever again, but I don't feel that as a loss because of what those foods did to me. Once I started with the sugar, it took me out of the experience, and all I wanted was "more." The event became secondary. I was no longer with the family, making memories and enjoying their companionship. Instead, I was just keeping company with the addiction.

I refuse to ever feel like I am missing out. Instead, my head is filled with gratitude that I no longer have to fight those demons. This positive focus makes the journey feel rewarding and helps sustain motivation.

Overall, mindset is the foundation upon which recovery is built. By fostering a positive, resilient, and growth-oriented mindset, individuals can better navigate the challenges of overcoming ultra-processed food addiction.

A strong vision helps you maintain motivation, especially when faced with temptations or doubts. It serves as a reminder of the larger purpose behind the day-to-day efforts. By adopting these mindset shifts, individuals can transform their approach to recovery, making it more manageable and sustainable. Mindset is the internal compass that guides actions, helps navigate challenges, and ultimately leads to lasting change.

The RFR Takeaways

How Positive Mindset Builds Health

It's crucial for us to recognize that creating a positive mindset isn't just about making ourselves feel happy. It's actually critical for our physical health. Various studies have linked an optimistic approach to life with improved longevity and reduced health risks in a number of areas.[2] It might even lower your cholesterol and reduce inflammation,[3] although we need to do further study to understand this in more detail. If it's true that improving your mental health can improve your physical health - and it certainly seems to be the case - then we've got a huge incentive to work on our mindsets and get into the "positive zone."

Some people wonder if it's really possible to change our mindsets. What if you feel like you were just born a naturally negative person?

The answer is that you can change your approach, although you do have to be prepared to put in the work, and it takes time and practice. Building a healthy mental muscle can require as much of a workout as building your other muscles; you need conscious, sustained effort, motivation, and determination. It's a challenge, but it's one with huge payoffs! Once you've strengthened your brain, it will be far more capable of supporting you in the tough times, just like any other muscle in your body.

How Can You Build Your Mental Muscle?

So, what techniques can you use to mentally train your brain? There are many options out there and different ones work better for different people, but we will share a few of our top favorites here for you to try.

---

[2] Topor, D. R. (2019, October 16). *If you are happy and you know it... you may live longer.* Harvard Health. https://www.health.harvard.edu/blog/if-you-are-happy-and-you-know-it-you-may-live-longer-2019101618020

[3] Solan, M. (2021, July 1). *Thoughts on optimism.* Harvard Health. https://www.health.harvard.edu/mind-and-mood/thoughts-on-optimism

Mental Reframing

When you're faced with something you don't want to do, how do you view that thing? Chances are, with dread. You might envision all the ways it can go wrong or think about all the reasons you hate it. That's normal, but it doesn't tend to make the situation better, and usually does the opposite. Fortunately, though, you've got the power to change that. Altering the stories we tell ourselves about the things we don't like can often mitigate the dislike and make it easier to handle the thing in question.

For instance, if you treat family events with fear because you know food is going to be a big part of them, you rob yourself of control and stop yourself from enjoying the event. Your focus is on the food - and remember, where thought flows, energy goes. You won't be able to stop thinking about the food, and you'll find it almost impossible to resist.

If you can change your focus and find positive feelings, the event is likely to go much smoother. Pick something else to think about! Maybe there's a cousin you haven't seen for years, or you can't wait to tell your funny work story, or you're taking a gift to someone and you're looking forward to seeing their reaction. Maybe it's something else. Whatever you choose to focus on, you'll find that it's much easier to deal with the hard if you focus on the positives. Remember, you're in control of where your thoughts go; you can make a situation feel great if you try.

You can often also aid your mental reframing by combining something you enjoy with a task you dislike. This is a great way to make the task feel more bearable and ensure that you do it. For example, you might save the latest episode of a show you love to watch while you're folding laundry, a great way to make the chore go quickly and ensure it's far less tiresome.

Embrace A Growth Mentality

First up, what is a growth mentality? It refers to our mental dialogue. A fixed mindset is where you believe that your abilities are fixed and cannot be changed. A growth mindset means that you have faith in your capacity to grow and learn new skills. It means that when facing challenges, you believe in your ability to rise and meet them, develop new strategies, and overcome difficulties. Indeed, you may even start to see challenges not as problems but as opportunities to prove to yourself your own strength, energy, and enthusiasm.

Adopting a growth mindset takes time and involves being conscious about how you view things in your life. When something goes wrong, take a bit of time to analyze your thought patterns. Do you jump to the worst conclusions or immediately assume you'll fail? How can you change that narrative to focus on problem-solving and positivity?

Be Patient

Many of us, when we decide to make a change, want it to happen overnight. We don't want to put in the hard work, we don't want to face the setbacks, and we don't want to wait for the results. We'd just like a quick outcome. That's why diet products and "hacks" to lose weight fast are so popular, but most of us also recognize that they don't work. To succeed, you have to be patient. You've got to be prepared for it to take time; you've got to be okay with not getting there straight away.

Anything worth having is worth working for. If you're consistent, you will meet your goals eventually. Patience will give you the resilience you need to weather the storms and hold on tight to the lifeboat when the seas are choppy, so don't underestimate how important it is. If you try to rush everything, the journey is just going to feel harder and so much more frustrating than it needs to be.

Focus On The Why

We've all got a reason for undertaking this journey. Often, it'll be about your health and your appearance, but it can also be about finding mental peace and a place of calmness and control. Whatever your "why" is, get it clear in your head and use it whenever you start to doubt your abilities. This is one of your most powerful tools in the fight against food addiction. It's what you can cling to in the hardest moments when you feel like you're slipping. It's also what you can use to pick yourself up after a setback. It's your motivator, and it will get you where you need to go as long as you trust it and let it guide you.

Define your "why" very clearly so that it's as strong as it can be. You might even find that it helps to write it down somewhere you'll see it regularly, so it becomes ingrained in your mind and helps you in the hard moments!

Treat Mindset As Mental Edits

Your mindset is essentially a series of mental edits that you string together to determine how you view life. Feelings are just thoughts, not facts. So, we can influence them through the art of mental reframing. This is really helpful because stress almost always exacerbates addiction. If we can control our stress levels, we can dial down our emotions and make them more manageable, reducing our risk of turning to ultra-processed foods. Remember that being calm can move you from "someone who struggles with food" to "someone who is reclaiming their health and well-being." This will change how you see your relationship with food, helping you gain confidence and feel in control. All of this can be done through the power of the mind, so edit out those unhelpful thoughts and start pasting in some positive ones!

Hopefully, those tips will set your feet on the right path so you can begin flexing your mental muscle and using it in this fight. Treat it like any other workout: you've got to put in the effort, and you'll see some amazing results if you do.

In the final chapter, we will look at bringing all of these different elements together so you can learn how to use them in a harmonious, powerful way that will let you make real changes in your life.

CHAPTER 10

Bringing It All Together

I n our final chapter, we want to talk about what brings all the different threads together for us. We've covered a lot of ground in this book, and here, we want to convey some final thoughts on community and the power of having support as you get onto the lifeboat. You're never going to be there alone, so what ties all the threads up neatly?

In essence, it's surrounding ourselves with people who support us, love us, and further our journey. We've already done a chapter on the importance of connecting to others in healthy ways, but there's a deeper level we haven't covered yet, which is what we'll look at next.

Jamie: The Power of Community

Throughout my whole recovery, at every stage from the very early days, community has remained a common thread that has kept me going. It has changed color and texture many times, but the thread has remained consistent and has been key to the progress I've made. It's what has kept me on the lifeboat when the sea is rocky and the waves are high.

I don't know if I ever really valued community until I began my recovery journey. I certainly had connections with my family and friends, and I loved them deeply, but my background meant that many of these were unhealthy and unsupportive, and I didn't really know what it meant to be in a space that was centered upon the opposite, where people were looking to help, heal, and nurture.

In my initial recovery, that all changed. A dietician that I connected with opened me up to a community of people whose lives didn't revolve around food but around a myriad of other activities. It was the first time I had experienced anything like that. It was a huge shift, and one on which my entire recovery centered. Without it, I'm not sure I would ever have reached the point I'm at today. Those early days of opening my eyes to the existence of other people and other focuses were the fundamental starting point for me, and it was from this community that I took my first steps. I began my healing process because I was powered by these connections.

The thread changed color as I found my way into a gym setting and met those who were focused on exercise. I realized what it meant to be wrapped in a world that was driven and goal-oriented, and it became a huge part of my recovery. I met some people who had been pursuing fitness for a long time and others who were at the very early stages of their journeys, like me. I marveled over the level of acceptance I found in that world, which had seemed so daunting from the outskirts. I remember the excitement of meeting them, talking to them, and learning from them. The next eight years of my life would be spent with them on my lifeboat, and as I gradually gathered experience, I learned brand new coping strategies and approaches. It was an enormously inspirational place to be.

I was also told I inspired some other people, which did wonders for my self-confidence, giving me the boost I needed to keep going. It transformed how I felt about myself and my journey toward fitness and health. It was unexpected and very cool, and it opened my eyes to the phenomenal power of being part of a community that cared. By 2015, I knew what community meant to me, and I knew how critical it was to my sense of well-being and growth. With that in mind, I began to intentionally create communities wherever I could.

It wasn't just about food or exercise, either. I joined local business development groups and mastermind groups. I tried to create connections wherever I went, whatever they were doing, even if it was unrelated to my life on the surface. I didn't actually join my first recovery community until 2017, but when I did, it blew me away. The growth and engagement in those communities were phenomenal, and I learned so much.

I loved being part of the group and learning from others, both those who had been around for a long time and those who were taking their first steps. I loved hearing their stories and exploring their journeys. I saw myself mirrored in their experiences and marveled over the similarities and differences. I felt like I had come home, like suddenly people everywhere understood me and grasped my struggles without me needing to say a word.

That led me into the 12-step world: recovery in many different dimensions. I attended meetings on alcohol addiction and drug addiction, even though I didn't have those problems. I attended sessions about relationships and communication. I sometimes had nothing at all in common with the groups on a surface level and possibly no experience with the subjects they were covering, but I still knew I needed to learn something from them, and I went along nonetheless. I immersed myself in the setup of communities and saturated my life with learning through connections.

I sat, listened, and absorbed. Even if the content wasn't specific to my life and experiences, the sense of community and bonding mattered to me hugely. I watched people stand up and expose themselves, becoming vulnerable. I watched others nurturing them and helping them. I then watched the roles reverse. The amount of trust could be astounding. Addictive substances and processes go beyond food and, for many, are intertwined. That is why it is a branch on our recovery tree.

The learning and growth in those spaces also amazed me. I soaked up information from these sessions like a sponge. I found similarities in all the differences. I learned more than I could have imagined was possible. I found the value of keeping an open mind and closing my mouth, listening, and taking it in. I also learned to look for common ground instead of focusing on divisions, and that made a huge difference in how I felt about the world and other people. We were more similar inside than I often thought initially. That realization was a wonderful way to drive back loneliness!

Over and over, I found myself being taught and re-taught the lesson that community was crucial. Whenever I started to feel frustrated and off-course, it was because I had lost my connection with others. If the threads broke, I spiraled. When the threads were strong and woven in with others, I was secure.

My spiritual community was another thing that added great richness to my life. It was a place in which I found an indescribably warm welcome. It kept me going when I traveled to New Jersey, alone and shaky after all my divorce, job loss, and other challenges. That's where I was first able to slot into a spiritual community, and I found myself welcomed with open arms despite my earlier reservations about religion. There were many people like me who had grown into their faith at later stages, and others who had been walking the path from the start. It didn't matter; we came from all over and joined together. We connected and bonded. It was the perfect setting for me to rediscover who I was under the trauma and loss of death and divorce. That community stabilized me at a very unstable time in my life, whether they knew it or not.

I don't always think of my spiritual community as being part of my recovery, but really, it's one of the cornerstones. It keeps my feet on solid ground. When I returned to Texas, I knew I needed a church that would offer me similar community groups, and I began to take part in any I could find. Taking the time to get to know people and learning about their lives, finding out about everything they've done and achieved, the ways in which they've changed is an indescribable and enormously inspiring experience. If they can do these great things, so can I.

In 2020, I found my way into another recovery group and, again, saw my progress coming along in leaps and bounds. I was able to give a lot and get a lot, and it was mind-blowing just what a difference that made to me. Even years into my recovery journey, there was so much I could gain from listening to others and from sharing my own journey. It was all virtual, but what an incredibly valuable experience! After the loneliness at the start of the pandemic, the difference it made was more marked than I would have thought possible.

Then Paige and I met in 2022, and we launched our podcast in spring 2023. We didn't intend to create a community at first. We'd just planned a podcast, wanting to help others learn from our experiences and feel less alone in the world, but very organically, a community sprang up from it within just a few months of launching. Perhaps it's because together, we realized the importance of connections... and so did those who were listening to our podcast! We are stronger when we join forces, so it makes sense that a community would open up from what we initiated.

We know that all of our members give to us, and we give to them. We value every person who invests their time in our community and shares their recovery process. Every single individual brings something new to our world and helps crystallize our understanding.

We were also amazed by who wanted to hear from us and how much response we got; a good lesson in not underestimating your own value, which is another thing that being part of a community teaches you over and over again! Our community has evolved into something incredible that we are enormously proud to share with others, and knowing the value that community has given me over the last couple of decades, it's almost unsurprising that it has taken this course.

Community has continued to be important to me in other ways, too. Following my encounter with the mold, you might not think that I'd be gaining support from others in the same way, since I'm not currently as active or working out regularly. However, the threads have continued to weave through my life, with support and healing coming from many different corners of the world to help me through this next challenge. At the same time, I've been drawing on all that I learned in the past from those many meetings and recovery programs, using the lessons, strengths, and stories that I absorbed then to fuel this next step of my journey. All the communities of my past still feed into my current life and are helping me cope with this new difficulty.

I know that as life continues and my recovery develops, the community will remain at the core of my experiences, like a linchpin at the center on which everything else turns. The threads are what hold me in place when the world spins out of control. Never underestimate the value of group experiences and the power of belonging. It's the key to success.

Paige: Collective Wisdom

As one of the leaders at RFR, you might think that I'm usually in a place of giving, not gaining. That's not the case! Something wonderful I've noticed about helping others is that you're often helping yourself, too. Nothing makes me feel more committed to my own recovery than taking someone by the hand and walking out of the depths of Hell together. It makes me want to be a better person when I see how hard our members are working. It gives me purpose, an important branch on our tree.

I recently heard about a woman completing the NYC marathon. Alone on the trail, she started to struggle (understandably) and not long after, she was passed by two men holding hands, one of them blind. To me, those men represent the epitome of community. The blind man was being enabled to undertake something that he could not have otherwise done alone. The leader was equally benefiting through his role. The immense amount of healing and sheer joy you get from giving is incredible. This is what we experience in our community on a daily basis.

I wasn't always aware of the power of community. Once, I was someone who thought they could do things just as well on their own as with others. Guess where it got me? Nowhere. Stuck in a cycle of restriction, binging, overexercising, and frustration. I stayed there for years before I found the power of community.

In my defense, I never knew support was available til my mid-50s; I found out about food addiction and support groups simultaneously. You don't know what you don't know! I just knew that when I started eating sugar, I couldn't stop. I was so grateful to learn that what was plaguing me was a normal biological response to an addictive drug. I didn't even know the phrase "food addiction" until this point.

Some people shy away from that phrase because they think it's somehow shameful. My question is, why? What did I do to feel shame? I have zero shame because I didn't do anything wrong, and now that I understand food addiction, I'm doing everything in my power to get on the lifeboat and help as many other people aboard as I can. That's where community comes in for me - a place where we can all help each other.

I had no idea of the consequences of sugar when it was first given to me - no child does. And it's not like I was out on the street trying to work a deal or score a hit. It was, and is, constantly in my face. Every birthday party, holiday, school activity, etc. My life suffered tremendously because of it, and it was only by finding a community that I found understanding.

Ultra-processed food addiction isn't widely recognized and comes with a lot of stigma, as we've established. A community provides a space where there is no stigma. Being surrounded by others who validate your experiences and understand the challenges can reduce shame and self-judgment, fostering a more compassionate approach to recovery.

Discovering a language for ultra-processed food addiction changed my world. Suddenly, I was able to find others just like me. I located a tribe, my tribe. It was a relief to know others had had my experiences, suffered in a knowing way, felt my feelings. Forgive the expression, but I felt like a kid in a candy store. I had found nirvana.

Before knowing of the concept of community, I did some individual coaching, and helped someone lose 100 pounds. She was so proud and felt like she could celebrate that Thanksgiving by allowing herself to have whatever she wanted. Before you knew it, that one day turned into several and she gained all 100 pounds back. I do not believe that would have happened if she were in a community of people supporting her, where she would have had a chance to check in and talk about what was going on. This is the type of misery and trauma I am trying to put a stop to through the efforts of Real Food Recovery. It's beyond painful to see people suffer.

A strange phenomenon occurs when you join a group of people sharing the most tender parts of themselves. It's like you're at a certain baseline and every share lets you bump up a few notches. You aren't just there to talk about your issues. When you listen to others problem-solving and working through struggles, you learn so many lessons. You find yourself rooting for them as if your own success was on the line. In turn, you know they have the same warm feelings for you. No one wants to see another suffer through this horrible disease. When you know how destructive it is, you don't wish it on your worst enemy. There is a sense of bonding in a community that can't be explained.

Community is also there for you in very significant ways. When I went on my first vacation attempting to be sugar free, I was determined to take everyone in my group along. During one of our meetings, I asked who wanted to go to Colorado and climb a mountain for summer vacation. Everyone's hands shot up. Okay, I was onto something here. I wrote everyone's names on a piece of paper, alongside "Sugar Free Vacation" in big, bold caps, then I folded it up and carried that paper in my breast pocket the entire trip. I took pictures and sent them to the group. We went to all kinds of places together, from tourist traps to the wooded forests, sending smiling photos after every stop.

That was phenomenal support for my first attempt to do something that seemed herculean. Not only did it make hard seem easy, but it actually made it into something to look forward to. Remember, if you aren't having fun in recovery, you're doing something wrong! This should be a pleasant experience, taking you from abstinence to abundance. Could I have done that vacation on my own? Maybe. Would it have been harder? Absolutely. Did I turn the task from drudgery into a happy experiment with friends? You betcha.

The bonding communities offer is also amazing. It gives you a sense of purpose, a feeling of belonging, a connection with those who can understand you better than anyone else. You can share anything with these people and they will understand. At RFR, we have that tight-knit feel. Everyone is cheering you on and loving on you when things get hard. It's a place of acceptance. You will be seen, heard, and understood. These are core human needs. When your needs are met, you feel safe, and you can start building self-trust and calmness. You can pull out of the trauma drive and relax. You begin to work *with* your recovery versus *on* your recovery.

Remember, connection is the opposite of addiction. Being surrounded by others who understand the struggles and share similar experiences can be incredibly comforting. It offers reassurance that recovery is possible. Whenever I leave a community gathering, a sense of hope washes over me.

I remember another key moment that hammered home the importance of community to me. I was standing in my daughter's pantry, playing the "will I won't I" game. It was pivotal because I was able to stop and ask myself, "How do I want to check in with my group tomorrow morning?"

I envisioned how the story would go and opted for the happily-ever-after choice, closing the pantry door with joy in my heart at the thought of sharing my success with my friends. Morning could not come fast enough. Wow, that level of accountability helps in those moments. It makes you dig deep into future-self thinking. It also means that if you have to reach out and say, "I'm in trouble and need help right now," you will have a swarm of people ready to help you through. Isn't it nice to know someone has your back and is rooting for you?! It helps sustain motivation when personal resolve wanes.

There's also phenomenal knowledge-sharing, of course, which speaks to the heart of a recipe queen like me. You might learn tricks that work for other families, get information about a new vegetable, or find out how others manage difficult moments. One of our members shared that to stay out of food during holiday parties, she has a seltzer with some cranberries, orange, and mint leaves. It lets her socialize and feel included, with no pressure to eat. It's such a great idea that I would have never stumbled across had I not been in a community!

There are many other advantages too, like having someone more experienced to help you navigate all your firsts. I've learned countless lessons this way. Once, I was dreading a family visit because of my food issues, and when the visit got canceled, I felt terribly guilty because I was happy. My leader at the time told me that early in recovery, those feelings were totally normal. She reassured me that as I progressed, I'd be better able to manage those situations, and it was okay to prioritize myself in that moment. She shared her own success story, letting me see what lay ahead if I kept working at it. That absolved me from my guilt, and allowed me to look at things in a new light. Had I not been in a community, I would have lost out on her wisdom. There are so many "aha" moments and so much enlightenment when you share.

There's also knowing that you have a soft place to land when something goes wrong. Every good community knows that relapses are common and can offer encouragement during these difficult times. I can't tell you how often my heart has been touched by the tears of someone hurting and how grateful I felt to be in a position to lift someone back up out of guilt and sorrow. Community members can provide positive reinforcement and remind each other that setbacks are part of the process, not failures. This support helps prevent one bad day from becoming a permanent regression, empowering individuals to get back on track without excessive self-criticism.

In a recovery community, everyone is striving for better health and emotional freedom from ultra-processed food. This collective energy can enhance motivation, making the process feel less daunting and more achievable. The communal effort creates momentum, letting individuals feel part of something bigger, which can be incredibly empowering. Even after initial breakthroughs, challenges may arise months or years down the road, and a strong community provides a continuous source of encouragement and guidance. Longevity in recovery is easier to maintain when people stay connected to a supportive network that understands the complexities of food addiction.

Having others walk alongside you on this journey helps to transform recovery from a lonely struggle into a collaborative, empowering process. Let's call it what it is: collective wisdom.

Key Takeaways

There's really only one takeaway that we want you to receive from this chapter, and that is this: You aren't alone on this journey. Perhaps you feel like your feet are on an empty path and everyone else is headed in a different direction, but it's not true. There are thousands of communities out there filled with people like you. You haven't done anything worse than they have done. You haven't felt lower than they have felt. Food addiction is an isolating experience, but we can change that by deliberately seeking connections.

Communities provide many things for people who are struggling, with the most important being a place where you can receive love, a soft landing when things go wrong, and a setting where you can hear hard truths in compassionate ways. Communities offer emotional support, accountability, shared experiences, and a sense of belonging. No one wants to feel alone in their journey, so take steps to find others you can connect with. Belonging to a group of like-minded people reinforces positive change and strengthens one's commitment to recovery.

Having a strong community to keep you on the lifeboat is what will help you bring all the other branches together. Food, sleep, movement, spirituality, stress management, connection to yourself and others, and finally, mindset. These are the things your community will help you nurture. Whether it's through knowledge-sharing, company, support, understanding, or just being a voice on the other side of the challenges, a community is often the true key to success in recovery.

If nothing else, by reading this book, you have become part of the Real Food Recovery community, even if your connection never goes any further! You are seen, heard, understood, and loved in more ways than you could know because you're walking a path with thousands of other feet and charting a course that we know seems impossible at times. We hope you feel us reaching out to you through our stories and words, creating a connection that you can keep in the darkest moments when the demons are particularly loud. We have faith in your ability to do this, and we hope that you can find a space - either ours or another - that nourishes you and brings you out of the tempest and into calm waters.

Conclusion

When we can't find the words, the body will speak. Through learning to listen to their internal signals, We developed RFR, a groundbreaking, revolutionary program to help others. The program uniquely addresses our recovery systems as a whole, which allows you to get back to a place where you can trust your body to send the right signals. The Tree of Life approach touches the major areas of focus, with the branches working together to form a beautiful, vital life where you can flourish and uncover your authentic self. There is too much to cover in-depth in one book, but we hope to have touched on several areas that resonate with you wherever you are on your journey.

It's a comprehensive, holistic approach that relegates food back to its proper place and puts it into perspective, reducing its emphasis and allowing you to balance your life more effectively. You may even find that as this process occurs, other areas that have slipped out of focus become sharper and more important again. You'll be free to raise your head out of the miasma of food and enjoy the rest of the world again. It's like coming up for air after being submerged in the water. That's the feeling we want to give to anyone who is suffering from food addiction.

RFR is a virtual, action-oriented recovery community that focuses on connection, growth, and belonging for all who are struggling with cravings, food obsession, and compulsive ultra-processed food behavior.

RFR Daily Connections is a community that promotes health, empowerment, and vitality. Through active daily participation, our members grow emotionally, mentally, and spiritually and become free from the chains of ultra-processed food. This is a place and time for our members to connect, share and receive personalized feedback on all their recovery conundrums. We provide individualized focus as members share their experiences and guide them into reflection. By focusing on their branches of recovery, each member uncovers what's keeping them stuck. From there, we empower each member with simple action steps to move forward.

We cover topics such as acceptance, thought life, love, relationships, self-esteem, triggers, travel, stress, restaurants, boundaries, addiction, cues, emotions, spirituality, obsession, forgiveness, movement, goals, intelligence, consistency, organization, body acceptance, substances, education, values, inner peace, family, environment, attitude, trust, and many more.

We also redefine success and work to make recovery fun! We make sure members have a game plan, an approach to tackle their difficulties, and we stress the value of progress over perfection. Our goal is to help you reach a state of calm, where food is peace and not chaos.

If you would like to join us in our lifeboat, our community would love to have you. We'll bring you into our world of understanding, where we celebrate the big and small wins, cheer each other on, and learn how to navigate the waves. We want to be your partners as you get your own lifeboat beneath you!

Find us online:

Website: realfoodrecovery4u.com
Instagram: @RealFoodRecovery
TikTok: @RealFodRecovery
Facebook: Real Food Recovery